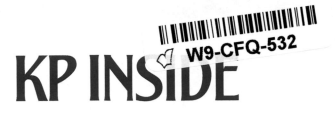

KP INSIDE

101 Letters to the People of Kaiser Permanente

GEORGE HALVORSON

6/20/2012

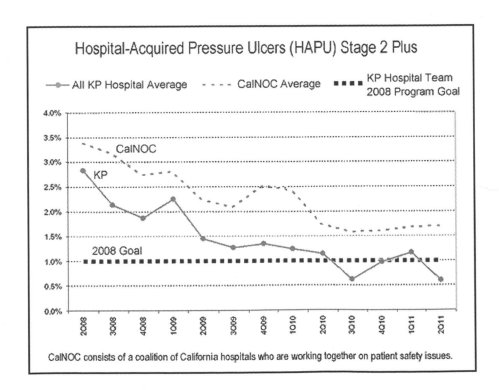

Hospital-Acquired Pressure Ulcers (HAPU) Stage 2 Plus

— All KP Hospital Average   - - - - CalNOC Average   ▪▪▪▪ KP Hospital Team 2008 Program Goal

CalNOC

KP

2008 Goal

CalNOC consists of a coalition of California hospitals who are working together on patient safety issues.

ISBN: 147.811.3669
ISBN 13: 978.147.8113669

Table of Contents

KP Letters – The Inside Story

Slightly over five years ago, I sent an email to our staff telling the 180,000 people who work and deliver care at Kaiser Permanente that I would write a letter to everyone on our staff every week for one full year. I told our folks at that time that I would personally celebrate something worthwhile and good about us every week for that entire year. I had about a dozen things in mind when I made that promise. I intended to stop writing the weekly celebration letters exactly one year from that date at letter 52. It turns out that I was actually wrong about stopping the letters at one year. I am still writing the letters every single week more than five years later. I continue to enjoy writing the letters and they keep coming off my pen, week after week.

The letters cover a lot of topics.

I write about KP successes — like reducing deaths from sepsis by half, or our groundbreaking Alzheimer's and autism research. I have written about our pioneering computer connectivity, our collective and collaborative diversity, and a whole series of other fun topics about various good things that we do. They are all letters about us, written for us and read every week by quite a few of us.

Other than taking one week off to get married, I have never missed a week in those five years. Even when I got married, I wrote a short letter that week celebrating both my marriage and my lovely new bride. Because my marriage was definitely good for my own morale as a Kaiser Permanente employee, I counted that letter as a relevant KP celebration. So if you include that letter, I actually haven't missed a single week in more than five years.

I do love writing the letters. I even love re-reading the letters. For me, writing those letters creates a lovely mindset. I am constantly looking for good things to celebrate. I definitely believe that I now know quite a bit more about us as an organization and as a care system than I would have known had I not been consistently writing these weekly celebration letters.

I do my own writing, so I write each letter myself. My letters and books are not written by anyone else. That isn't a chore for me because I love to write. I also learn when I write. These letters help me learn very useful things about us every week. So I believe that writing all of the weekly letters would have been a good use of my time, even if I hadn't distributed them to anyone else.

I do have help with the letters.

Many people offer ideas for letters. That is good and useful input, and it is much appreciated.

I always have our legal people and our data and quality people review every letter that I write to make sure that whatever I say runs no risk of being factually wrong. Being accurate is a particularly good thing. I love being right — and I have learned over decades that it can take a team effort to be consistently right.

The internal readership for the letters tends to be fairly high. People at KP often talk to me about the letters. Many of our staff call them "Be Well" letters — because I end every letter suggesting that people "Be Well." People frequently offer thoughts or comments or insights about specific letters. I get quite a few email responses to most of the letters, and that email feedback has been both reinforcing and educational. Sometimes those response emails from readers trigger individual follow-up by me. I often get pointed to a new letter topic by those responses. Sometimes I learn things about us from those emails that would otherwise have not been known or visible to me.

So why am I now telling the background story about these letters and why am I now turning 101 of them into this book? For starters, I like writing books. I have written several books. I enjoy writing books — and this has turned out to be a remarkably easy book to write. So that's one reason to turn all of these letters into a book.

Another reason to write this book is that I have had a number of both external and internal requests for reprints and redistribution of several of the letters. This book is an easy way to make some of the most requested letters easily available for re-reading.

Several outside readers who have had a chance to read some of the individual letters have said to me, "I had no idea that Kaiser Permanente was doing the work you described in that letter."

I hear that a lot, actually. We do a lot of things below the radar screen of the outside world.

So it seemed to me that it might be a good idea to share a number of the letters more broadly, to let people know we are doing the work I discuss in these letters. One hundred and one is a purely arbitrary number. I liked the sound of it as a subtitle for the book, and it forced me to be a bit selective in my choice of letters. It was actually a wee bit painful to cut some of the letters that I cut to get down to 101 total letters for the book.

To make the letters in this book more useful and easier to understand for outside readers — and because I love to write about these topics — I have written a short tee-up note for many of the letters. I hope the tee-up notes put the letters themselves into better context so they will make more sense to people who do not work for Kaiser Permanente.

The letters, themselves, are untouched. I only changed one part of one letter for this book. I did correct one error in one letter that I missed earlier when I sent out that letter. With that exception, these letters are exactly what I have written to the people of Kaiser Permanente every Friday afternoon for more than five years — printed here exactly as written each week.

This book isn't a textbook. It isn't an official organizational position statement. It has pieces of history in it, but it isn't a history book. The letters are not legal documents and they are not formal training pieces. This is a simple book of letters. The letters are what they are — letters to the People of Kaiser Permanente, written by someone whose job is to help facilitate, support, and celebrate the good things we do and who has chosen the weekly letter format to do some of the celebrations.

My day job, when I am not writing letters or books, is to be the CEO of one of the most interesting health plans and hospital systems on the planet. It's a great job. At Kaiser Permanente, we are responsible for the care of nine million people. We are a care system. We take care of patients and we deliver more than 50 billion dollars in care every year. Our almost unique dual role and combined accountability for both care delivery and care coverage gives those of us who work at Kaiser Permanente a melded perspective about care delivery that may be useful and even thought-provoking for a lot of people who think only about either the delivery of care or the financing of care. We do it all — and we have to think about all of the pieces all of the time. That is a really fun perspective and one that can be useful to people who are focused just on the pieces of the care problems and the care opportunities.

The very first letter that I include in this book is the very first weekly letter I wrote to the people of Kaiser Permanente nearly five years ago. That first letter makes a set of basic points about hospital safety and process improvement in care delivery that I have echoed many times in the letters that followed that first letter over the next five-plus years.

That letter triggered a ton of great responses. Hundreds of our employees wrote email responses to me after that first letter. Most of the respondents to my first letter were delighted to learn that we were doing this particular quality improvement work and doing it in the way we were doing it. A number of the email responses asked questions. Many offered suggestions. That letter created a nice dialogue on those issues. The volume of responses and the contents of the notes and the pure energy in the feedback told me immediately that writing the weekly letters was probably a good idea.

So this book begins with the actual Celebration Letter Number One — enjoy.

Celebrating My Very First Weekly Letter – September 27, 2007

Dear KP Colleagues,

The charts below are something we should celebrate. They are definitely a win.

Both charts are from Northern California. The first chart shows a year-over-year increase in the number of our hospital patients with pre-admission pneumonia who received the full set of seven recommended treatment approaches while they were in one of our hospitals.

Hospital Composite of Pneumonia Treatments: 2005 - 2006

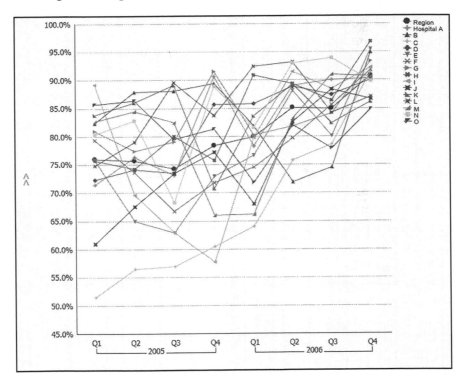

The second chart shows the improvement in processes aimed at preventing surgical procedure infections.

Hospital Composite of Surgery Infection Control: 2005 – 2006

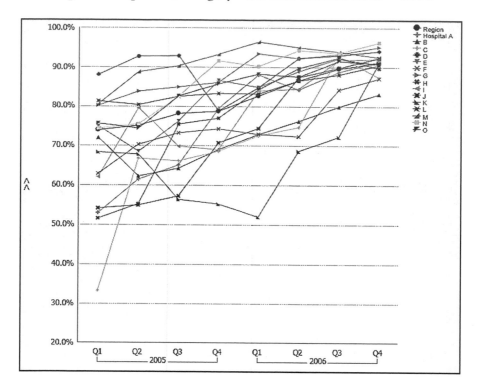

Both charts demonstrate important work. The charts show that we were able to improve and extend the level of care for our hospital patients. Patients are getting more complete care, and our care levels are doing what we want them to do.

When I was speaking to the National Governors Association a couple of weeks ago, I shared these exact charts with them, and they interrupted me with applause.

Why did they applaud? Because we made people's lives better. They applauded because in each case, we obviously identified a problem, measured the problem, focused on the sources of the problem, and then took steps together as a team of caregivers to fix the problem.

Data was an essential first step in that process. Without data, this level of care improvement cannot and will not happen. Our hospital leaders and key physicians literally did not know what our hospital-specific numbers were for the total package of recommended care for those infections and processes in 2004. We treated our patients well everywhere and we had an extremely high level of compliance with the top priority treatment steps everywhere — but because we started measuring these processes, we now know that we did not provide the full and complete set of recommended treatments every time, everywhere. We measured that composite performance for the first time in 2004, and then we shared that information with each other in 2005 and 2006. Improvements resulted.

I know for a fact that our hospitals who were at the very lowest performance levels on each of these charts did not know that to be true in 2004. Everyone thought in good faith that we were doing a good job everywhere. But when we measured and knew what our real hospital-specific scores were, then opportunity was created and we started down the path to real improvement. Look at the numbers on these charts. The worst performing hospitals in January of 2005 were among our best performing hospitals by December of 2006. That performance continues to improve.

I told you in my letter last week that I intended to celebrate a Kaiser Permanente achievement as a success every week for a year. This is my first note of celebration. It reflects a job well done — and an absolute commitment to do even better.

So thank you to the physicians, the quality leadership, the hospital leadership, and to all the caregivers in each of the hospitals who made this happen.

I love these charts. It shows what we can do. It also shows very clearly why data matters. Without the actual data, that lowest scoring hospital on each chart would have simply assumed in good faith that they were doing a complete job — and, I suspect, the 2007 approach for each hospital would have been the same as the 2005 approach. That is obviously not good enough for us as a community of caregivers who care about the care we deliver.

So well done, Northern California.

As I said in my letter last week, I intend to celebrate a success every week. Hundreds of people wrote to me after my last letter. I am still responding. Some of the responses will take a bit because I need to look something up or hunt something down. That is happening. But I do want to hear from you this week. Is this weekly letter a good approach? What is your reaction to this week's topic of "celebration?" Let me hear from you.

Be well,
George

✿ ✿ ✿

Background Note: Sepsis Kills More People than Stroke or Cancer in Hospitals

We are one of the largest hospital systems in the world. We know from years of actual experience at Kaiser Permanente that safety for each hospital patient depends on hospitals doing the right things and doing the right things consistently and well. It is our job as caregivers to figure out where care can be made better and safer, and then it is our job to do that work.

One of our major themes for our care improvement agenda has focused on sepsis. As the next two letters show, sepsis is the number one cause of death in American hospitals. Sepsis kills more people in hospitals than stroke, heart attacks, or cancer. Most people do not know that to be true. We have taken systematic steps in our hospitals to reduce the death rate from sepsis significantly. We did that work because our members and our patients trust us with their lives. They deserve us doing this important work and doing it well.

The most recent sepsis letter says that America could save 70,000 lives a year if everyone in every single American hospital did what we have now learned to do.

Celebrating Our Sepsis Mortality Reduction Successes – November 18, 2011

Dear KP Colleagues,

Sepsis kills.

Sepsis is actually the number one cause of death in hospitals in California.

According to the official state death rate statistics, more people die in hospitals from sepsis than die from cancer, stroke, or heart disease.

State statistics tell us that 24 percent of seniors who die in California hospitals — nearly one in four seniors — die from sepsis.

Very few people know that to be true.

Very few people are doing anything about it.

Our goal is to have the safest hospitals in America, so we are an exception to that rule. We are doing something about sepsis — and what we are doing is working.

In fact, if you look at the charts below, it's easy to see how well we are doing.

When we started measuring the percentage of our sepsis patients who did not survive, our first mortality numbers were significantly more than twenty percent.

One in four sepsis patients did not survive.

Now we have made consistent improvements in every hospital and our death rate has dropped to eleven percent.

That is half as many people passing on.

The chart below is from a research paper we published showing the world how to improve sepsis care. That chart came from a pilot program.

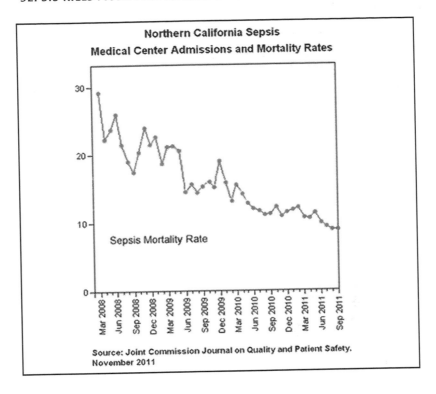

The second chart shows the results for all of our hospitals. We learned from our pilots and we are now succeeding in all of our hospital sites.

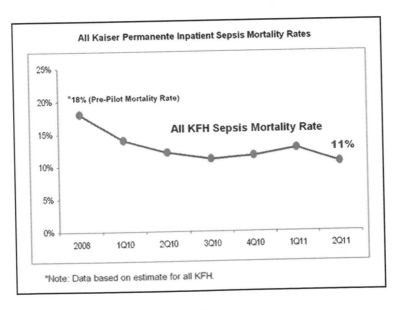

The second chart shows the average for all KP hospitals. Some are now less than eight percent.

How did we do that? How did we save all of those lives?

We had very smart people focus on the problem to figure out what we needed to do to make care better for sepsis patients.

It turns out that speed is essential. There is a time called the "Golden Hour" at the beginning of treatment for each patient where rapid intervention with the right treatment really is golden.

Delayed care can be fatal. Fast care can work miracles.

So we figured out how to diagnose quickly, pre-plan every response, predefine the right medications, and train people in our care sites to respond in a hurry with the right stuff in the right way.

Most hospitals — outside of KP — usually do not have sepsis response teams or even organized sepsis treatment plans.

In too many other hospitals, just getting the blood test results back to the floor where the patient is waiting can take hours. Ordering medications in those other hospitals can take a long time, and the medication can take hours to get to the patient.

Inventing a sepsis response from scratch for each patient is the wrong way to deliver care for sepsis patients.

In our hospitals, we have teams of nurses, pharmacists, lab techs, and physicians all knowing that getting sepsis care right for each patient may be the most important thing that ever happens in the life of that sepsis patient.

It is literally a life and death situation. We save lives because we work in teams of caregivers focused on saving each of those lives.

It is incredibly important work. For the person who doesn't die because we get it right, it's hard to imagine anything more important.

I had written a letter earlier to share some of our initial successes with sepsis care. The good news is that our successes are continuing. Continuous improvement is a celebration all by itself.

We are now sharing our learning and processes with the rest of health care. We are working with a national coalition — Partnership for Quality Care (PQC) — to spread our learnings to some of the best hospitals in the U.S.

PQC hospitals are setting a goal of reducing sepsis deaths by at least twenty-five percent. I believe they will all succeed.

We are also publishing our learnings in research journals sharing what we know with the whole world. The Joint Commission Journal on Quality and Patient Safety just ran an article on our sepsis treatment successes. That first chart came from that article. More than thirty-five news media outlets ran stories about that research paper.

The article is extremely important because it tells the world not to surrender to sepsis.

We did not surrender to sepsis.

We did not say — "Sepsis happens and that's too bad."

Instead, we said — "Sepsis happens — let's save a lot of lives by responding really, really well to provide the right care to every patient."

That's the right answer.

So my letter this week celebrates the brilliant teams of KP folks who figured out how to save all of those lives — and all of the caregiver teams who are getting better at saving lives every day.

Continuous improvement is a wonderful thing.

Well done.

Be well.

George

✲ ✲ ✲

Celebrating Doing the Right Thing for the Right Reasons in Sepsis Care – April 20, 2012

Dear KP Colleagues,

Sepsis kills.

Sepsis kills more people in California hospitals than stroke, heart disease, or cancer.

We have been focused for several years on the mission of reducing deaths from sepsis in our hospitals.

Very, very smart people at Kaiser Permanente have done very good work. We have learned from each other, applied the best science and applied the best processes, and we have done that work with great consistency.

The chart below shows our success rate. Our caregivers are doing really great work and doing it over and over — every single day.

The chart clearly tells the story.

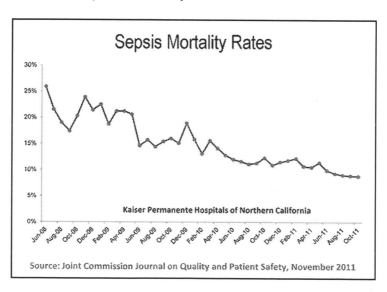

Every single KP hospital is now doing better than just about any other hospitals at sepsis care. We don't know who does a better job — but we do know that if other hospitals improved their sepsis care to the level we have achieved, that would save 70,000 lives a year in this country.

That means 70,000 American families who would not have lost a loved one to sepsis last year. This really is important work.

I have written about our sepsis care successes before. So why am I writing about them again this week?

I am writing again because I just received a letter from one of our sepsis patients. The letter reminded me again very clearly that we are here for people — for the members and patients and families we serve. Sepsis results are important numbers at one level — but sepsis results represent actual people at another level, and it is the people we help that counts more than numbers.

I thought I would share the letter. I removed the name from the letter — but the person who wrote it gave me permission to share it. This is the real story of a real patient, and it tells a truth about the total experience of being a sepsis patient that numbers can't convey.

Even with survival, recovery can be hard. Survival alone is not the whole story for a sepsis patient. Getting back to functioning from a bad sepsis infection can be about as hard as surviving the first onslaught of the infection. So treating it early is really important because early treatment means much less sepsis damage.

This particular sepsis patient is a double one of us — she is a KP patient who is also a KP employee. Here is the letter:

Hello,

As I read stories about the support Kaiser Permanente provides within health care, community, and operations, I realized my story relates to all. I work for Kaiser.

A few years ago I was struck down by double pneumonia and became septic within days. I thought I had a bad flu. I was in the fight for my life and began to know it as I saw the x-rays and test results in the ER (I worked as a Respiratory Therapist years before). After three days, I realized I was losing the battle and was in amazement, witnessing my body going into painful multiple-system failures, and thought, "So this is how dying feels."

Miracles began to happen. As my body let go, I felt an unusual loving strength start to flow into my being. My co-workers sent messages, notes, cards of hope and prayers. After seven days, I was moved out of the ICU and onto the floor for another seven days. My doctor told me, "People generally don't make it with so many organ system failures. It is very special to see you here with us."

My legs had stopped working while in the hospital. So upon returning home, I made a point of creating a collage on my closet door of all the beautiful notes and best wishes from my co-workers. Every morning, I opened my eyes to see all the hope and prayers lit up by the morning light. When I got a new card, I made myself walk across my room to post it. I went from a wheelchair, to a walker, to a cane.

Months later, I was able to return to my job. My first days back I ended up in a wheelchair, and my co-workers took turns getting me back and forth in the office. This positive support and hope was and continues to be tremendous in my recovery.

Last year, I had major surgery, due to my previous health event. Again, KP remained encouraging and supportive as I recovered.

I am challenged with many health issues, and without the outreach from my Kaiser providers helping me to find my way and try every aspect of care to improve my quality of life, I would be lost. I will begin a pain management course next week that I am very excited about. But my message today is my gratefulness towards my work team. My Kaiser supervisors and my co-workers have connected me with HR and every other tool needed to figure out how to keep my professional world intact and go above and beyond their job duties. I wish there was a reward for such recognition. They are a large part of the saving grace I experience daily. I just wanted you to know one of the amazing stories happening within our Kaiser doors.

Thank you for taking time to read my story.

That is the letter I received. Sepsis isn't just about numbers. Sepsis also isn't just about survival. Sepsis is also about recovery, and sepsis is about people. Sepsis can have a huge negative impact on people's lives even when the patient survives.

So the work we do to intervene early and to reduce the damage done for each patient is incredibly important.

We need to become even better at doing that care well because real people are affected in very real ways for a very long time.

My letter this week again celebrates our sepsis response teams. Thank you for the work you do every day. More than 70,000 Americans in other care settings would not have died last year if they could have had the care we give our patients with that infection every single day.

Well done.

Be well.

George

✿ ✿ ✿

Background Note: Pressure Ulcers Also Need Our Attention

To make our hospital patients safer, we have also focused some of our best and brightest care team members on the prevention and treatment of pressure ulcers in our hospitals. Pressure ulcers are nasty things. They disfigure and kill people. They can be a truly horrible experience for the patients who get them.

The next three weekly letters about pressure ulcers speak for themselves. As do the results.

Making care better for pressure ulcer patients is a complete labor of love. It is a labor of love because the work starts fresh with each and every patient and there is no down time relative to doing what needs to be done to keep those ulcers from damaging people and even destroying people's lives.

Nurses do miracles for pressure ulcer patients. Great nursing care saves lives and keeps lives from being ruined.

That's why we need great nurses who can spend their time with patients instead of spending their time doing paperwork and administrative functions.

Helping nurses spend time on patient care instead of spending time on paperwork was the subject of another weekly letter. The next three letters are about pressure ulcers and best care.

Celebrating Major Reductions in Hospital-Acquired Pressure Ulcers – September 10, 2010

Dear KP Colleagues,

Hospital-acquired pressure ulcers happen far too often.

I have been involved in the direct operations of hospitals for a couple of decades now. In the old days, when pressure ulcers happened, people said, "Oh Dmmm — another one. That's sad. But I guess that's just what happens to some people who spend time in hospitals."

It was actually both really sad and unfortunate that for a very long time, way too many really good people who delivered care even in great hospitals just accepted those ulcers — and the pain and the deaths that sometimes resulted — as being a "normal risk" of being hospitalized.

We simply called those problems "iatrogenic," and that generic and semi-technical label somehow almost served to remove a level of accountability from hospitals for those cases. "Iatrogenic happens," was the belief for a very long time.

We are a lot smarter now. We know that a very high percentage of those ulcers can be prevented.

We know that our patients' lives are a lot better when those ulcers are prevented.

We know very practical and consistent things that we can do in our hospitals to prevent many of those ulcers from happening.

When you put all of those pieces together, what we get is a Kaiser Permanente initiative to actually prevent as many of those pressure induced ulcers as we can.

We are not perfect. We are far from perfect. But we are making progress, we are continuously learning, and we are committed to making care better for the patients in our hospitals.

Hospitals should be a place of safety for each and every patient who has to be there.

We want our Kaiser Permanente hospitals to be safe, and we want the people we care for in our hospitals to both feel safe and actually be safe.

So how are we doing on hospital-acquired pressure ulcers?

This chart shows how we are doing through the first quarter of this year.

The top line on the chart isn't just us. It shows the average pressure ulcer level among patients in a regional collaborative of over 200 hospitals who measure those events. The lower line on the chart is us, and it shows our total Kaiser Permanente ulcer levels.

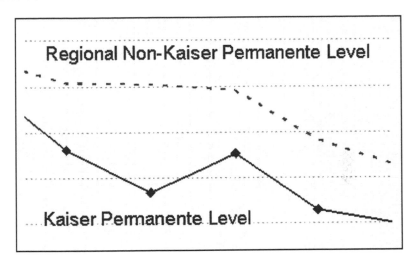

We are making measurable progress.

We have significant numbers of very real patients who are ulcer free today who would have had pressure ulcers without our program. Their lives are definitely better because we are doing what we are doing.

We did not make that progress by wishing it would happen. We also didn't make that progress by giving pep talks or sending out memos about ulcers.

We made that progress because really smart caregivers figured out real-world process improvements that our care teams could use in a consistent and focused way with our patients who are at risk of those ulcers, and then we actually made those improvements happen.

Consistency is golden. Being consistent with best practices saves lives.

Look at the chart. Lives are being saved. Ulcers are being avoided.

So my letter this week celebrates the really smart and practical caregivers who figured out what we needed to do to prevent those ulcers and — even more importantly — my letter celebrates all of the caregivers and care teams at Kaiser Permanente who care so much about the well-being and safety of our patients that the things we need to do for our patients' safety are being consistently done — over and over again — for each patient in our care.

If any of us were in the hospital, it is exactly what we would each want for our own care.

Be well.
George

✡ ✡ ✡

Celebrating Our Pressure Ulcer Prevention Program – December 17, 2010

Dear KP Colleagues,

Pressure ulcers can eat through the skin and muscle of a patient and create a wound that is all the way to the bone.

Pressure ulcers can disfigure patients, sometimes forever. After ulcers heal, plastic surgeons often have to repair the damage caused by the ulcer in its destructive stages.

Pressure ulcers can kill — and it can be a very painful way to die.

Pressure ulcers have been a major curse of hospital caregivers for as long as hospitals have existed. Every hospital has its truly sad stories about patients whose lives were ruined and ended by pressure ulcers.

Why am I writing about pressure ulcers and the misery they cause in my weekly letter?

We had our annual Dr. David Lawrence Patient Safety Award ceremony on December 1. Every year, we celebrate a region that has done an exceptional job on patient safety.

This year's winner was Northern California, for putting in place a pressure ulcer prevention program so effective that two of our hospitals went two full years without a single reportable Stage 3 or greater pressure ulcer.

Zero is an amazing number.

Zero takes an incredible consistency of caring for each patient. Zero is the result of care so good it deserves to be called deeply compassionate care — treating each patient like family — taking the patients' best interests so much to heart that every single patient gets the care they need to make sure those ulcers don't happen.

We have a video that was done for the award dinner showing the care teams who put that wonderful program in place. You can see the video on our Quality website.

I urge you to watch it. You will see that our caregivers are a team — focused as a team on each patient who needs us to get that care right.

Caregiving is a 24/7 commitment.

There is no coasting in hospital care. There is no down time. We don't get to get a great score on a quality report, declare victory, and go back to doing other things.

Each patient needs us. The patients we have today need us today — right now.

There is immediacy to great care and there is a loving consistency to great care that makes great care something we achieve and then achieve again, and then achieve again.

Preventing pressure ulcers is a wonderful thing to do. The patients who never get a Stage 3 or higher ulcer don't know how extremely lucky they are to be getting their care from us — because we care enough to make sure those ulcers don't happen.

The attached chart shows how our overall pressure ulcers reduction program is going. We don't have all of our hospitals down to zero reportable ulcers, and even with the very best of care, some ulcers will happen, but we are making very good progress across all of our hospitals and our goal is zero. You can see from the chart that our hospital regions, overall, are doing better than the other hospitals who also measure those ulcers and work to prevent them as well. And we are doing a lot better than the hospital systems or sites that have not made pressure ulcer prevention a priority for best care.

So my letter this week celebrates our Lawrence Award care sites who have zero reportable pressure ulcers, and I am also celebrating our overall agenda, for all regions and all KP hospitals, to make those ulcers the rarest of adverse events for the people we serve.

Congratulations. Well done.

Watch the video if you can.

Be well.

George

PRESSURE ULCERS ALSO NEED OUR ATTENTION

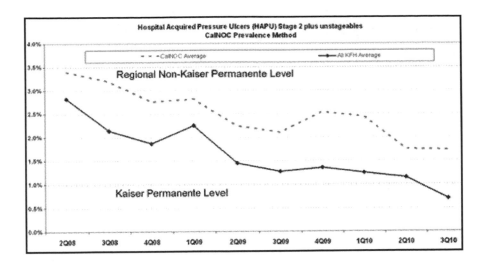

✿ ✿ ✿

Celebrating Our Reduction in Hospital-Acquired Pressure Ulcers – December 15, 2011

Dear KP Colleagues,

Every hospital in the world has patients who suffer from pressure ulcers.

When those ulcers happen to a patient, life can get very grim. Patients can be in great pain. And many pressure ulcer patients end up permanently disfigured and sometimes functionally impaired.

Some patients die.

It is very much not a good way to die.

We took a look at our own pressure ulcer rates in KP hospitals a couple of years ago. We measured ourselves to see how many of our patients were getting pressure ulcers.

The answer for us was 2.8 percent. Slightly fewer than 3 percent of our patients were getting those ulcers at a stage 2 or higher level.

Two-point-eight percent is not a big percent. But when we have three dozen hospitals that are each serving a full array of patients every single day, 2.8 percent still means that a lot of people were going through the misery and the pain and the damage of having those ulcers.

We wanted comparative data to see if 2.8 percent was a normal rate for pressure ulcers.

We looked around to see how well other hospitals were doing on that issue.

Data about pressure ulcers was not easy to get. We were lucky and we found a coalition of hospitals in California who shared our concern about hospital-acquired pressure ulcers. Those hospitals were tracking the ulcer rates and many were working together to bring down their own pressure ulcer levels.

How were they doing?

They were then at 3.5 percent of their patients suffering from those ulcers.

So the good news was that we had colleagues and allies in the hospital world to learn from and to compare success with. We also learned from their data that our 2.8 percent was not the worst rate for those ulcers. It was a good number by comparison with those other hospitals.

So what did we do next?

We could have just celebrated the fact that we were doing better than other concerned hospitals on that measure.

We did not choose that approach. That's not who we are.

We owe our patients great and safe care.

People join us as a health plan and as a care team and they put their lives in our hands.

So instead of celebrating the fact that our numbers were better than some other care sites, we brought together some of our brightest and best people to figure out how we could do significantly better than we were doing.

We set a goal.

The goal we set back in 2008 wasn't to cut pressure ulcers in half. We aimed higher. One percent. We actually set a 1 percent goal. Our goal was to drop the number of stage 2 and higher pressure ulcers to less than 1 percent of our patients.

One percent is a world-class goal.

One percent means that a lot of people will not be damaged by those horrible ulcers.

It isn't easy to bring down the rate of pressure ulcers.

Reducing pressure ulcers is hard work. Extremely hard work. It is work that is never finished.

It starts over and over with each and every patient.

It takes great nursing care to get to 1 percent because most of the work done with each and every at-risk patient requires superb nursing skills, and nurses who care enough to care well and deeply and care skillfully for each and every patient.

It's also a team effort. Physicians, nurses, and other caregivers are all deeply involved — and it is a team effort that never lets down because when each healthy patient leaves our hospital bed, a new patient moves into that bed, and that new person needs us to protect him or her from those ulcers.

It is a labor of skill, competence, and even love.

So how are we doing?

We are making a difference.

The chart below shows our success rate on preventing pressure ulcers since 2008. It also shows the success rate of the other California hospitals in the Collaborative Alliance for Nursing Outcomes (calNOC) coalition that had the 3.5 percent ulcer incidence rate back in 2008.

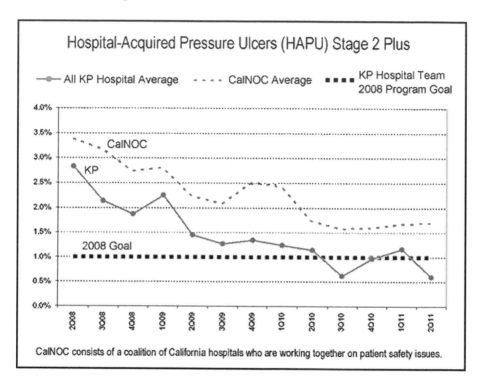

We, however, have actually now dropped our pressure ulcer rate in our hospitals below our 2008 1 percent goal. Our hospitals have worked together, learned from each other, and we are now at a level no one believed possible when we started this journey of continuous improvement a couple of years ago.

We are now under 1 percent.

We are now down to six-tenths of a percent of our patients who have a stage 2 or higher pressure ulcer.

Six-tenths of a percent is a lot lower than 2.8 percent.

We actually now only have one-fifth as many of our patients at that level compared to our levels when we started down this road in 2008.

In this holiday season, celebrating all of those people who trusted us with their care and did not have to go through the misery of having a pressure ulcer and who are now home with their families is a good thing.

So my letter this week celebrates both the very bright and committed people who built this process for KP and who have continuously improved it — making us functionally better and operationally smarter every day — and my letter also celebrates the people of Kaiser Permanente who are in each room with each patient multiple times every day looking for each risk situation and caring for each patient at a very personal level. Our care teams and our caregivers deserve to be celebrated.

It's all about people. People caring for people.

We have won some external awards for our hospital care. Those awards and external recognitions are good — but they are not remotely as important to us as achieving our own goals of protecting our patients and delivering the right care. No one is perfect. But we are making progress that we can and should all celebrate.

Well done. This chart tells a story we can all be proud of. The world is a better place both because we are doing this work and because we are proving it can be done. And our patients are in a better place because we are who we are and because we do what we do.

Be well.

George

✳ ✳ ✳

Background Note: Preventing Pediatric Hospital Infections is Particularly Good to Do

We have reduced sepsis deaths, central-line infections and pressure ulcer levels in our hospitals. All of those programs have been focused primarily on adult patients. That is a good thing to do — but the truth is, we also need to address those issues for kids. Kids can get infections in hospital settings, as well. For obvious reasons, the very smallest kids in the hospital can be the most vulnerable.

So my letters about Pediatric Intensive Care Unit infections have also focused on an important patient safety issue. We have done a lot of work to reduce overall hospital-acquired infections. We are particularly proud of some of the work done for kids.

The next letter celebrates some of that work.

Celebrating PICU Safety – October 10, 2008

Dear KP Colleagues,

When adults acquire post surgery or inpatient infections, the results can be tragic.

When children in pediatric intensive care units get infections, it can feel even more tragic.

Children have fewer defenses and very small children have very small internal reserves, and the kids can die or be permanently damaged by those kinds of infections.

Preventing those infections in our smallest patients is an act of mercy and an act of real caring.

So this week, I am celebrating star performances by two of our Pediatric ICUs.

The Sacramento PICU (pediatric intensive care unit) has gone a full year without a single VAP (ventilator associated pneumonia) or a single central line bloodstream infection (CLBSI).

Our Santa Clara PICU has gone the last four quarters with only one VAP and also had zero central line bloodstream infections.

The national CDC (Centers for Disease Control and Prevention) benchmark level for PICU BSIs is currently 5.3 infections per 1,000 central line days. Their equivalent benchmark for PICU VAP is 2.5 infections per 1,000 ventilator days.

Five bloodstream infections or two cases of pneumonia doesn't seem like very many — unless you are one of those children. And then life can be painful, hellish, ugly, and very sad.

So, zero is a lot better. And we are now proving that zero infections can be done, if we take every systematic and careful step needed to protect those children.

My own newest grandson just finished three months in a NICU (neonatal intensive care unit) in Pennsylvania. He was born at 2.9 pounds and he just went home from the hospital at five pounds — so that is a very good thing. While he was in the hospital, another baby in a nearby care unit ran into bad times. That was not a good thing. Problems in those units can be horrible for the parents and even worse for the child.

When you are a parent or a grandparent, you really appreciate having caregivers who take the extra steps to make your child safe. You appreciate caregivers who think zero is the right goal when it comes to infections and then do the very careful care steps needed to make zero infections real.

So congratulations to the heroes at Santa Clara and Sacramento Medical Centers who kept our children safe.

Well done.

Be well.

George

✻ ✻ ✻

Background Note: Preterm Births Can Create Their Own Tragedies and Issues

One of our great strengths as a total care system is that we can take the long view on a topic, and we can make changes in a systematic way that have an impact across a broad spectrum of patients. As other letters in this book point out, we have done that work successfully across the entire continuum of care for heart care, diabetic care, broken bones, HIV treatment, cancer detection and treatment, and a wide range of care agendas.

How do we make a difference? For one thing, we look at the total process of care for each health care problem.

Our preferred approach is to go upstream on the total care process for each disease to achieve maximum impact on behalf of our patient. Actually preventing broken bones is a brilliant and proactive way of dealing with broken bones, for example.

For our kids, there are very few areas where we can go upstream more effectively than to focus on reducing the number of premature births — for obvious reasons. This letter also gave me another chance to write briefly about one of my own grandsons — the tiny little one who was born very prematurely.

Preventing preterm births is a wonderful thing to do. We have put some very effective programs in place at Kaiser Permanente to actually reduce the number of premature births. Kids who are born prematurely often face more difficult health issues for their entire lives. Reducing premature births saves lives and — for many kids — significantly improves their entire lives.

The next letter celebrates some of our success levels in reducing the premature births levels with solid and systematic prenatal care.

Celebrating Our Neonatal Care Teams – September 5, 2008

Dear KP Colleagues,

We had 2,800 preterm births last year in Northern California and 3,030 preterm births in Southern California.

If we had the same number of preterm births as the state average for our population, we would have had 4,545 preterm births in Northern California and 4,208 preterm births in Southern California.

The very best way of lowering the number of preterm births is to make sure we deliver great prenatal care to our members who are pregnant. Better care in the months prior to birth make a real difference in the likelihood that pregnancies go to full term.

Preterm births can be highly traumatic. Sadly, in some cases, the outcomes are tragic.

So reducing the number of preterm births is something that we need to do well.

That whole area of care is one that is particularly important and meaningful to me right now because my newest grandson was born one month ago in Pennsylvania at the heroic size of two pounds and nine ounces. Today, a month later, he has grown to three pounds nine ounces. He is now drinking from a tiny bottle, breathing without an air tube, and his father (my oldest son) was just able to hold him yesterday for the first time.

When a baby is that small, tiny victories are huge victories. Taking a first bottle or keeping breathing going without interruption for more than two hours on end is a kind of miracle.

So we are all feeling good about the progress that he is making. We are having daily celebrations and we are literally counting and sharing each ounce of progress.

Usually, data like the total number of preterm births in our system are a statistic — a measurement — a way of judging volume and activity and progress. Sometimes, however, when the relevant number is just one preterm birth, the statistic becomes incredibly immediate and very, very real.

So this week I am celebrating all of our caregivers who take care of our preterm babies — and all of the OB care team members who keep our overall preterm birth numbers so low.

I am also celebrating — for all of us who have had the personal blessing of achieving that special status — Grandparents Day.

This Sunday is Grandparents Day.

Enjoy. I am.

Be well.
George

✡ ✡ ✡

Background Note: Successful Reductions in Hip Fractures

Kaiser Permanente is a full spectrum provider of care. We are responsible for the total health and care needs of nine million people. That full scope of responsibility does give us a different perspective than most care sites. We aren't just focused on waiting for patients to be sick or injured and then providing pieces of care to mitigate the damage. As I said in my weekly letter about reducing the number of preterm births, we really do want to actually proactively reduce the need for multiple categories of care for our patients. We work particularly hard to anticipate, prevent, and mitigate future care issues for our patients.

Our goal is to solve future health problems for many patients by actually preventing specific health problems for each patient. We believe strongly in strategic and functional interventions — not just creating incidental clinical reactions to individual clinical crises. Many of my weekly letters celebrate our successful interventions that change the level of care needed by patients in a good way.

One area where we have invented very effective interventions that have had a huge impact on patient care is in the area of broken bones. Other care systems simply treat broken bones; we prevent them.

The next letter was also one of the very first ones I wrote. It celebrated a very effective program and care strategy that is now a hallmark and pioneering victory for preventive care for seniors and a model for the country across all of our care sites.

Preventing broken bones is a good thing to do, as this letter celebrates.

Celebrating Our Healthy Bones Program – November 7, 2008

Dear KP Colleagues,

Hip fractures can make life very miserable for anyone who has one.

They hurt. The fracture makes people immobile. It's definitely not a good situation to be in.

When your hip is damaged, you can't move easily or without pain. The healing can take a long time, and the surgery that is sometimes needed has its own universe of discomforts, annoyances, miseries, and risks.

So why am I writing about hip fractures in my weekly letter?

I am writing because our pioneering "Healthy Bones" program in Southern California has reduced hip fracture rates by more than 37 percent in over 620,000 people. That's a lot of hips that aren't damaged.

I expect that this will very quickly become another set of learnings that is shared with non-Kaiser Permanente patients through both the news media and professional publications.

For some folks at risk for osteoporosis, we have cut the risk by 50 percent.

How did we do that?

By being proactive.

By being systematic.

By focusing on prevention — and not just treatment.

Just about everyone else in health care waits until the patient is damaged and then provides remedial care. Other care organizations generally specialize in waiting until a patient's hip breaks and then they try to fix the breaks.

We prevent the breaks.

Why don't others prevent the breaks? Partly because the economic model of most health care is so flawed that almost no one even funds research or supports studies that focus clearly on prevention. The sad truth is that there is no business model for fee-for-service orthopedic hospitals to support prevention research. So that research is very hard to find.

We believe in prevention. We believe in good health. We use our available resources to figure out how to help people avoid fracturing their hips. Each of our regions has a Healthy Bones program and they all work. Southern California is my focus for this letter because we just finished measuring the results of the Southern California program, and our researchers are now publishing an article to share what we have learned.

Our Southern California caregivers have solid data that tells us we made 37.2 percent of those fractures disappear.

There are more than 300,000 hip fractures every year in the US. If other care systems used our approach, 100,000 or more of those hips would not be fractured.

Prevention is a wonderful thing. Other studies have shown that half of the people with hip fractures never regain their old functional capacity. Twenty five percent of elderly patients with hip fractures actually die in the first year after the accident.

So we have learned how to use a combination of bone density tests, anti-osteoporosis medicines, and patient education in a consistent, standardized, science-based way to make those fractures less likely to happen.

We use KP HealthConnect® — our electronic medical record — to aid the Healthy Bones team with the identification, risk stratification, and tracking of our osteoporosis patients. Other care systems also don't have KP HealthConnect.

We will be sharing what we have learned about preventing hip fractures with the world.

It's the right thing to do.

So my letter this week celebrates our Kaiser Permanente of Southern California "Healthy Bones" program — and all of the "Healthy Bones" care teams across Kaiser Permanente.

People's lives are better with healthy bones.

Be well.

George

✳ ✳ ✳

Background Note: Data Registries on Focused Topics Can Really Lead to Better Care

We love data. We love looking at facts and learning about care. When your search for the truth about patient care is supported by real data about patient care — and when that data exists in viable quantity and is focused on real care — the learning opportunities can be golden.

We believe that to be true. We actually know that to be true. We provide care to 9 million people — and we are responsible for maintaining the medical records for those 9 million patients. We have computerized all of our medical records — with the largest private medical record success levels in the world — so that whole array of computerized data can now be used in multiple ways to improve care.

Having all of that patient data in computers creates a lot of opportunity for learning. It also, functionally, creates a wonderful amount of information. We love using our data to figure out how to deliver better care and to make better decisions about care.

The next letter celebrates one effective use of real patient data — our joint replacement registry. We probably have the best repository of information about joint replacements in America. We have a great joint replacement registry because we have chosen to keep and collect that information, and we have chosen to be a learning organization. The approach we are using to study the data and improve care using the data is becoming a model for the country, and we are currently helping other care sites in this country build a national joint registry agenda.

The next two letters speak for themselves.

Celebrating Our Total Joint Replacement Registry – September 3, 2010

Dear KP Colleagues,

Our computerized registry of total joint replacements now contains information about more than 100,000 joint replacements.

That is by far the largest database on hips, implants, and related surgeries in the country.

We have used that database to figure out what works and doesn't work. Our physician research team adds to our own data a constant scanning and review of other good hip and joint research to help our 350 Kaiser Permanente hip surgeons deliver really well-informed care.

Other folks have written lovely and complimentary articles about our data tool. More than 130 newspaper articles and media stories have been written about our registry just this year.

People wrote those 130 news stories because quite a few people outside KP know that our registry works to improve care, and they know it works well as the core and basic data set for important research into replacement surgery.

If those were the only uses and benefits, our Total Joint Replacement Registry would be a huge win.

But that's not all our registry does. It also lets us find specific patients who need additional care.

Why would patients need additional care?

The New York Times wrote a story just last week about Johnson and Johnson having major FDA-level complaints about a hip replacement implant made by their orthopedics subsidiary.

J & J has now withdrawn the product from the market.

So what did we do with that information? In total, across all of American health care, there were about 93,000 of those particular J & J hips implanted.

We did 622 of them, affecting 557 of our patients — as some patients had both hips replaced. That is the bad news.

The good news is that our computerized patient registry told us which of our patients received those hips. We know the patients. We are their surgeons. So we will now do our own follow-up to see what the results have been for our own patients — and we will figure out which of our patients need our help.

Hip surgery is not fun for patients. It's a hard thing for a patient to go through the surgery and the rehab. Going through that whole painful process twice, because your first hip implant failed, is even less fun.

Worst case is not being a Kaiser Permanente patient and having a hip that is problematic and being lost as a patient in the total unorganized health care information infrastructure because no one knows you are a person who has that problematic hip, and no one is programmatically accountable for tracking your progress and status and helping you deal with those issues.

They are not having an easy time finding the other 93,000 patients. We have found ours.

So the good news is that we have the tool to help when bad joints happen. And we are helping.

Our Total Joint Replacement Registry is a great asset for care delivery.

So my letter this week celebrates all the people at Kaiser Permanente who had the brilliant idea to create the Total Joint Replacement Registry and then did all the hard work necessary to make it real and keep it running.

Well done.

Thank you.

Be well.

George

✻ ✻ ✻

Celebrating Another Vohs Award
Winner – January 25, 2008

Dear KP Colleagues,

One of the great deficiencies in health care in America and in the world is the lack of good and valid comparative information about what works.

New technologies spring up in health care all the time — and no one tracks the results of those technologies over time to see how well each approach works.

One reason for that huge deficiency in follow up is that the people who manufacture a given drug or prosthetic device generally have no economic motive to actually compare product effectiveness. If they do a comparative study and their product turns out to be less effective than someone else's product, that definitely could be bad for sales.

People in those businesses don't very much like to do things that are bad for sales.

So, the truth is that patients and consumers in the health care world need someone to do that work — to record data, track outcomes, and make comparisons.

We will be giving out two "Vohs Awards" this year. I wrote last week about the superb CCCS heart program in Colorado, with a 73 percent reduction in coronary artery disease mortality. That program was one Vohs winner for 2008.

The second winner is a different but also very important program called The Kaiser Permanente National Total Joint Replacement Registry (TJRR).

Almost no one in the United States really keeps track of large numbers of total joint replacements. We do. A team of orthopedic surgeons, chiefs, orthopedic clinical staff, operating room staff, orthopedic department administrators in Northern California, Southern California, Hawaii, Northwest, and Colorado, and our National Infection Control staff have put together what might be the largest set of reports and follow up on joint replacement in this country.

47

We not only keep track of joint replacements, we take steps to improve the quality and outcomes of our own joint replacements.

If you are a patient whose leg has been cut open so surgeons can insert a large mechanical foreign object into your body, you will go through pain, discomfort, and extensive rehabilitation that will, for a while, dominate your life. Then, if things go as well as they should, you will walk again and pain will not be how you define walking across a room or climbing a stair. That's the goal. But sometimes there are problems. For a number of people with a joint replacement, infections set in — or the joint doesn't set right — or the process somehow falls short. When that happens to you as a patient, life isn't as good as you would like it to be. So as a patient, we each want our caregivers to have the highest possible success rate and we want the implants to last as long as possible.

That's the goal of the TJRR. The process tracks outcomes. It measures results. It keeps track of how many times particular approaches and devices work or do not work.

That whole process is being linked into our new KP HealthConnect® system and it is teaching that system how to add value relative to a procedure based area of medicine. This is new work for KP HealthConnect. We are currently learning how to do that work — and that is an extremely important thing for us to learn because very few people other than us have enough volume to build comparative data about surgical procedures and implants.

So what are we learning? Let me share one chart with you as an example. One set of comparisons was done by the TJRR team based on the category of cement used to hold the new joint in place. Approaches vary. Some patients had a basic cement, some had a hybrid cement, and some were uncemented — a technique favored by some manufacturers. Until we did the study, no one knew whether there was any difference in the survival time of the implanted joints based on the cement approach used. It turned out that there was a measurable difference, as you can see on the chart below.

No solo doctor working from the experience base of a small and single medical practice could ever uncover that level of joint survival differentiation. The number is big enough to make a difference in some patient's lives but it is far too small to be detected from a few dozen cases done by a single doctor or by a small practice. For our doctors, care patterns changed when that data was learned and shared. Fewer patients needed second implants. Data combined with shared learning made a difference in patient care for the people who didn't need to have to have the surgery done twice.

So this week, I am celebrating our TJRR team — the 300 surgeons and 50 hospitals who contribute to that data base and make care better. We now have data on over 55,000 total joint replacements in our system.

Well done — and thank you to our Total Joint Replacement Registry team.

Be well.

George

* * *

Background Note: Patients With Multiple Health Conditions Need Team Care

The next letter celebrates another innovation success that helps us deliver team care. Across all of America, 75 percent of all health care costs come from patients with chronic conditions. Roughly 80 percent of the costs in this country come from patients with co-morbidities — multiple health conditions. In most care settings, multiple health conditions mean multiple doctors who are usually not connected with one another in any way. In the rest of the country, the separate doctors who treat each patient usually do not exchange care plans, and usually they don't even exchange basic care data about the patients they share.

That is sad. It is also ineffective. In many cases, it is dangerous. Patients with multiple doctors need their doctor to be a team. We have built-in team care at Kaiser Permanente. We start as a team. We have now increased our effectiveness as a team hugely by having electronic medical records with all the data for every patient. A single blended electronic medical record for every patient shows each care team member for each patient all care data in real time for each patient. We do team care better all the time because we make team care a goal, and we support the team care process with the right tools. We build the tools to do the work — rather than building the work around the tools.

My next letter celebrates the kind of care that happened when we did super-focused team care for a targeted group of our high-need patients. We decided to very carefully focus intense team care on a set of patients with triple co-morbidities. What happened as a result of that focus? Care got even better — and, as you can read in the letter, we ended up cutting the need for hospital admissions for those patients by more than half.

Team care works. Team care has been the subject of many of my weekly letters. Again — this very early celebration letter on that topic to our staff speaks for itself.

Celebrating Hawaii Care Results for Special Patients – November 26, 2008

Dear KP Colleagues,

Hawaii is making major progress on some key areas of focused care improvement.

Our Hawaii Region just celebrated its 50th birthday. We had a series of talks, meetings, parties, remembrances, public events, private events, employee gatherings, and a month long campaign of public education and community service.

I had the pleasure of staying again in a hotel built on Waikiki beach at the approximate site of our first Kaiser Permanente hospital in Hawaii. Henry Kaiser had a wonderful sense of location.

The Hawaii care team made a number of presentations about our care delivery achievements in Hawaii, as part of the celebration.

One of those presentations featured a pilot program created in Hawaii to take advantage of our new electronic medical record. The goal was to figure out how to focus our care on a set of patients who need care most.

This particular pilot took every single patient we had in Hawaii with the "deadly trio" of co-morbidities — congestive heart failure, coronary artery disease, and diabetes.

Patients with any one of those conditions need a lot of medical support. Patients with all three of those conditions really need us to help. The "triple burden" patients go through frequent, painful emergency room visits with depressing regularity — and the triple burden patients are often hospitalized.

Being hospitalized with a heart attack is never something to look forward to.

Being hospitalized with congestive heart failure may be even worse. As a patient, you are drowning in your own body fluids. Air pipes and fluid drainage pipes run down your throat.

It's painful, uncomfortable, sometimes very frightening, almost always life threatening, and generally quite unpleasant.

Avoiding those kinds of events is a good thing if you are a patient. A very good thing.

So how did we do when we focused on our "triple-burdened" patients?

The Hawaii care team did a superb job.

By focusing on each patient through a doctor and nurse support team, systematically doing all of the follow-up needed for each patient, monitoring each of the patients closely, and educating each of the patients about their own likely early symptoms of an imminent crisis, our care team cut the number of hospital admissions for those patients by over 65 percent in just six months.

That's a much better quality of life for our patients. Lower hospital admissions also takes some pressure off our hospital beds and helps us focus on incident prevention rather than incident response.

I was equally impressed by the fact that the proactive, system-supported, care team approach in Hawaii cut emergency room visits for those same patients by 34 percent.

That's actually another fairly major improvement in the quality of life for those patients. No one likes to go to an emergency room as a patient. Emergencies are almost always unpleasant episodes in our lives, and we tend to be better off when they don't have to happen.

So any processes that can reduce emergency room visits by one-third and also reduce crisis-level hospital admissions by two-thirds is a process that we as patients should deeply value and appreciate and we as caregivers should deeply respect.

Well done, Hawaii.

Congratulations on fifty years and congratulations on being at the leading edge of our collective efforts to learn how to effectively use and build on the new systems and databases that we have built. No one else in health care has ever had this resource. We are the first — and we are learning what it can do for patients and for care delivery. Hawaii is taking a lead role. Patients are benefiting. Lives are better.

Well done.

It's a time of thanksgiving for those patients — and it's now a time of Thanksgiving for us all.

Be well — and have a great turkey day.
George

* * *

Background Note: Improving Both Accuracy Levels And Safety At Shift Change in Hospitals

As one of the largest private medical groups in the world and one of the largest hospital systems in America, we are constantly looking at ways to improve the processes of care delivery.

One of our most successful care delivery innovations involving team care at Kaiser Permanente happened in our hospitals. This approach was a brand new idea for us and it was new for the entire world when I wrote the next letter way back in November of 2007.

We very carefully reengineered the way we transfer information from care team to care team when shifts change in hospitals.

That may seem like a simple and obvious task, but it is very important work and it generally isn't done.

Hospitals run 24 hours a day, seven days a week. There are usually three full teams of people needed to keep hospitals running each day. So hospital shifts tend to change every eight hours. When shift change happens, the people who delivered care in the old shift need to share information about each of their patients with the caregivers in the new shift who will now be responsible for those patients. We discovered in our own hospitals that that information-transfer work for our patients at shift change was not being done consistently from site to site and unit to unit. We also discovered that some significant communication errors happened far too often at shift change and these errors could put patients at risk. That wasn't acceptable to us — so we did some very nice process redesign work to reduce both of those problems.

The concept and the process we invented for improving information transfer at shift changes that is described in the next letter has since become a national standard, and the Joint Commission on Accreditation of Healthcare Organizations (JCAHO) now refers to our shift-change, information transfer process as a best practice for the hospital world and has endorsed it for other hospitals. Most other hospitals do not have a formal information process at shift change and still have the kinds of challenges and problems we had before we changed our process.

The November 2 celebration letter way back in 2007 tells the story of how we systematically made shift changes safer and more effective.

Celebrating Nurse Knowledge Exchange – November 2, 2007

Dear KP Colleagues,

So what are we celebrating this week?

Competent, consistent caregiving...when shifts change in our hospitals.

Most people do not know that one of the most "dangerous" times to be in any hospital can be at shift change. All hospitals take care of patients 24 hours a day. That means — if people work an eight hour day — that every hospital needs three separate shifts of people to provide 24 hours of patient care.

Continuity of care is essential for each patient. So it is important for the people on the current shift to inform the people on the incoming shift about the needed information for each patient.

That information exchange process takes time...an average of 44 minutes per nurse, per shift. During that information exchange time, patients sometimes decide to go to the bathroom or cross the room on their own. Patients have described the time period during shift change as a "ghost town." During that time, hospital caregivers are exchanging needed information, not spending as much time with patients.

There are a couple of obvious and significant potential problems with that entire shift-change process in most hospitals. One problem is that it does take time away from face-to-face patient care. Another problem is that almost no hospitals completely structure or fully choreograph the data flow for the process, so the quality and accuracy of the specific information flow for any given patient often depends on the judgment, memory, and thoroughness of the two caregivers involved for each patient. Everyone wants to do that job perfectly. Every single caregiver wants to do exactly what patients need. But people can be tired after a long shift — and people can be eager, impatient, and even slightly less focused at the beginning of a shift. So the information transmission process at changes of shift can sometimes have inaccuracies — omissions — errors and misunderstandings — or temporary, incidental memory lapses.

Remember the old classroom game where you whispered something to one person, who whispered it to the next person, who whispered it to the next person, etc? Remember how garbled that information flow could get in just a few transmissions?

Verbal transmissions of patient information from shift, to shift, to shift, to shift have some risk of these same kinds of distortions.

Why am I writing about that somewhat negative point of process misfunctionality in my weekly celebration letter?

I am writing about that topic because Kaiser Permanente almost uniquely has addressed those exact problems head on and we have done something about them. Remember, we are caregivers. We own and operate hospitals. We take care of patients. We definitely care about our patients. We think about ways to improve care. This was an opportunity to do exactly that. We knew what those shift change information exchange problems were because just about every hospital in America has them.

So what did we do?

We had frontline teams of nurses, administrative staff, physicians and other caregivers led by KP's own Innovation Consultancy team spend time to figure out a better way of getting that essential information passed accurately, consistently, and efficiently from caregiver-to-caregiver, shift-to-shift.

Our teams from all of our hospital regions did wonderful work. The teams designed a great information exchange process that involves getting the same exact and complete set of data communicated very consistently between caregivers at every shift change.

In what I believe was a stroke of pure genius, our caregiver teams also moved the location of the process. The data exchange moved from the sometimes distant nursing station at the end of the hall into the patient's room — and made the patient part of the information exchange when the patients are awake and available to join in the process.

Templated whiteboards and computer systems were both designed to support the new process.

The total time needed for a nurse to see her or his first patient was reduced from 44 minutes to 12 minutes. The "ghost town" effect was eliminated. Accuracy was significantly improved. Patients felt more involved — and actually were involved where appropriate. (We don't wake patients up to do the process.)

We prototyped the approach in several care units, and then we piloted it in those hospitals with our frontline nursing staff. It has been a huge win. So we now have rolled it out to all of our shifts at almost all of our hospitals. The remaining couple of hospitals are scheduled for implementation in the near future.

Other non-Kaiser Permanente hospitals generally still rely heavily on a less thorough, less accurate, less patient-friendly, and less efficient process.

We are choosing a different path — a better path — a collective and collaborative path — and everyone should benefit. So this week, we are celebrating the people and teams of caregivers that made all of that care improvement happen. Outside organizations have also recognized us for that innovation, so I am not the first to celebrate that success. Our Nurse Knowledge Exchange program has already been featured in the Wall Street Journal. Descriptions of the process will be included in several books, including the Ten Faces of Innovation by Tom Kelly, Spreading Improvement Across Your Healthcare Organization by Kevin Nolan and Marie Schall, and Improving Hand-Off Communication by Joint Commission Resources. The Nurse Knowledge Exchange program is also listed in the Agency for Healthcare Research and Quality (AHRQ) Innovation Exchange Database.

As a side note, you may have noticed that I have not been naming individual people in my weekly celebrations of performance improvement. Let me explain why that is true. I have not been naming specific people because each of those efforts has so many heroes. I am concerned that if I list any names, I will omit someone who really deserves to be mentioned. This particular shift change effort had obvious pioneers, heroes, advocates, champions, supporters, and enablers at multiple levels. Rather than miss naming any involved or deserving person, I am using this letter to thank all of the teams and not naming each of the relevant names.

Please give me your feedback on that approach. Should I name more names even though I may not get them all listed or should I celebrate the specific achievement and generically thank the people who were the heroes who "achieved" without naming them individually?

What do you think?

In this particular case, re-engineering our hospital shift change process, we definitely do have many real heroes. You know who you are. You did a great thing. Thank you.

And be well.
George

* * *

Background Note: Medication Errors in Hospitals Can Be Reduced

Another major process improvement achievement that I have celebrated in a couple of my letters relates to things we have done to reduce prescription drug errors and adverse events in our hospitals.

Experts tell us that there are nearly 400,000 preventable drug related injuries in American hospitals every year. Across the country, we know that prescription drug errors in hospitals cause about 7,000 deaths a year.

We knew that some of these errors and some of those deaths have happened in our sites. So how are we dealing with that reality?

We have actually focused on that issue in multiple ways. One of our more innovative efforts to address that problem is celebrated in the next letter.

Celebrating KP MedRite – May 16, 2008

Dear KP Colleagues,

Credible experts believe that there are between 380,000 and 450,000 "adverse drug events" or ADEs in American hospitals every year.

The Institute of Medicine estimates that those ADEs cause about 7,000 deaths every year. Why would that happen? Why would hospitals in America make so many medication errors that 7,000 people who should have been going home to their families instead go to a mortuary and a funeral ceremony?

Those errors are never intentional. They are accidents. They are often mistakes made because the caregivers had incomplete or inaccurate information about the drugs they were giving to patients.

Knowing that those numbers are true everywhere in American health care, we knew they had to be true for us as well.

As caregivers who care deeply about our patients, we have had very capable and competent caregivers working on reducing our own internal error rate.

In an earlier letter, I talked about changing the size of our pill bottles for some medications and changing the available doses for others — to significantly reduce the likelihood of us making those ADE errors. Those are all good projects and approaches that we are building on and they are in sync with best practices of other American hospitals.

My celebration this week is about a very innovative new approach that is — at this point, unique to us — called KP MedRite. It's an approach that isn't intuitively obvious. It resulted from having our innovations team and front line nurses working together to look at the whole process of medication distribution to figure out when and where in the process errors were more likely to happen.

In analyzing that situation, it turned out that a major cause of errors was having the person dispensing the medication distracted while doing the distribution. Distractions happen all the time in the process of care delivery. Patients need care. New information arrives for caregivers. Emergencies happen.

So what happened in the care delivery redesign process? The goal was set to prevent distractions for the nurses who distribute medications.

How could that be done? The team came up with a really clever idea. The nurses with the medications started wearing brightly colored sashes over their uniform while dispensing medications. Everyone else in the clinic or hospital was told that no one should distract or even interact with a nurse wearing the protective "zone of non-distraction" sash.

That approach worked. It made a real difference. The nurses with the sashes were able to focus exclusively on the task at hand — getting the right meds to the right patient at the right dosage at the right time.

Other elements of the new medication safety plan involve creating a quiet zone around the Pyxis drug dispensing machine and setting up sensor lights that let people outside a medication room know that a nurse is inside preparing meds.

The approach works. We are expanding it across our care system to all of our hospitals. It's a best practice that safety organizations outside of Kaiser Permanente are beginning to notice. I expect within a year, we will see our idea becoming a norm in many other hospitals around the country. The Joint Commission on Hospital Accreditation asked us to write it up and submit it to the Joint Commission as a possible best practice for all hospitals.

So congratulations to the nurses in our care sites who pioneered this new approach to make lives better — and longer — for our patients.

Across the country, 7,000 people are dying every year from ADEs. Yellow sashes might cut back on those deaths significantly.

One additional piece of advice — if you are in a KP hospital and see a nurse wearing a brightly colored vest or sash, don't distract that nurse in any way. Important work is being done. Appreciate the task and stay clear of the process.

Have a good week.

Be well.

George

* * *

Background Note: Hospitals and Clinics Are Not Our Only Sites of Care

We have done a lot of innovative things with the design of our clinical spaces and our hospitals. I have celebrated some of those care site innovations and developments in my weekly letters. We are redesigning our sites of care.

We are also experimenting with new places and new sites of care. We are being innovative in designing in-home care and in creating remote access e-care. A number of celebration letters have talked about our leading role in using both computers and smartphones as a care delivery support tool — sending lab results to patients and setting up email visits with our doctors.

In between e-care and traditional clinical care, we are also experimenting with "mobile" care. We are now delivering some care from medical vans that can bring real technology to mobile patient care sites. A couple of my celebration letters have dealt with our new Mobile Clinics. We now have several of the new high functioning vans in different sites. The Hawaii experiment described in this letter was a success. Our new high tech care vans can be brought to various work sites and even to schools and community centers for on-site care.

We pioneered that approach in Hawaii — as this first celebratory letter on that mobile care topic describes.

Celebrating Mobile Care – July 10, 2009

Dear KP Colleagues,

A minister blessed one of our buses last week. Technically, it was a van. A million-dollar mega van that we built to serve as a mobile clinic for a Hawaiian island that does not have enough care sites. The Big Island of Hawaii has a spread out population, expensive gas, very few care sites, many one-lane roads that can make travel time consuming and difficult, and we have over 22,000 members.

Our KP Hawaii team realized that it might be easier to bring care directly to our members on the Big Island rather than bring members to our care.

So our team invented a mobile care site that can move around the island on a regular schedule.

The Mobile Health Vehicle (MHV) may be the first of its kind in the world. The vehicle has 500 square feet of electronically supported health services on 10 wheels that will begin next week to bring care to our members across the 4,000 square miles of the Big Island.

The MHV will be staffed by a Kaiser Permanente nurse practitioner, a medical assistant, and a mammography technologist, and we will have physician services available as appropriate for various times and places.

This team will be able to provide basic exams and screenings, including cholesterol, colorectal, glucose, waive testing, urinalysis, and gonorrhea and Chlamydia testing. Flu shots and pneumovax vaccines will be available.

And of course with mammography equipment and a mammography technologist on board, mammograms will be available. We plan to provide an average of 28 mammography screenings per day, or 5,200 visits per year. This is a huge number for an island where mammography screening rates are now well below both state and national averages.

Lives will be saved because of that service.

One key difference between our new MHV and other types of mobile care equipment is that we have Kaiser Permanente HealthConnect® linked directly to the vehicle. Members will be getting our electronic care support services and our connectivity brought directly to them.

The MHV team will be fully connected to KP HealthConnect with real-time update capabilities. And, to fill out the care continuum, video consultations with specialists are also available from the vehicle.

It's a very well-connected vehicle.

We will not only do mammograms on the MHV — we will do them with state-of-the-art digital mammography technology, thanks to our KP-IT team. We will be learning how to stream the mammograms, which means that the mammograms will be transmitted electronically and will be read remotely. Our own IT folks are developing a technology that is, we believe, the first in the nation — transferring mammography images in real time to our radiologists across the water at the Moanalua Medical Center.

I had a chance to take a personal tour of the vehicle when it stopped in Oakland a couple of weeks ago for a final inspection. I love it.

We are a continuous learning organization. So we will learn a lot from using this MHV. We are already exploring new services to add to it. I expect that a year from now, we will be even smarter in figuring out how to move care around on wheels. So that is my celebration letter this week. I am celebrating our new mobile health vehicle, and all of the KP people that turned the vision of a caregiving vehicle into a mobile reality.
Be well.
George

✿ ✿ ✿

Background Note: We Want All the Right People to Get Their Flu Shot

We love prevention. We love continuously improving our prevention agendas.

Flu shots are a great preventive tool for the right people. So we work very hard to get all of our senior patients immunized.

We also have target lists of other people who need the shots — and we work hard to connect with those high-risk patients to get those shots done. We want to immunize everyone — and we particularly want to immunize the folks that need that prevention the most.

Flu shots lend themselves, surprisingly, to innovation. The old model of going to the doctor's office and getting a shot as the sole focus of a one-to-one patient/caregiver contact is a good thing — but that approach isn't sufficient if we really want a lot of people to get flu shots in a very short time frame.

I have now written a couple of letters about the various fun and creative ways we help members get those shots. We actually held the Guinness World Record for the most flu shots in one site in one day.

That was another letter. This early celebration letter deals with drive-thru flu shots that we have set up in multiple care sites. One of our primary goals as a care system is to "Make The Right Thing Easy To Do." These efforts help us achieve that goal.

Celebrating Drive-Thru Flu Shots – November 21, 2008

Dear KP Colleagues,

I was in a meeting the other day learning about some interesting and creative things that we do, and one of our staff members said that the single most creative thing her own clinic did was convenient flu shots — and she, herself, was the direct beneficiary.

I've seen flu shots in work sites, hospital lobbies, parking lot portable vans, and pharmacy waiting rooms, so I thought I already had some sense of the broad spectrum of needle-insertion opportunities.

"What made your flu shot so special?" I asked.

"I didn't have to get out of my car," she said, "My medical center does drive-thru flu shots. I drove up, rolled down my window, stuck out my arm, and got my shot. It was a huge time saver for me."

That seemed like a really good idea, so I checked on the site. It turns out that we have quite a few sites where members can get their flu shots without unfastening their seat belts.

Most are in covered parking ramps or under awnings, so they are protected from bad weather.

At our Richmond, Northern California site, we've become so efficient that we gave over 3,500 shots — or nine a minute — on the first Saturday of flu season, to people sitting in their cars.

The Bay Area sites average over 3,000 patients a day early in the season and the numbers drop down to 1,000 a day by season end.

In Orange County, we immunized over 13,000 people on October 18 and over 9,000 people on October 25 in three drive-thru sites.

In South Bay, we have been doing drive-thru sites for 10 years — and have done 2,500 immunizations in a single day.

We also do drive-thru shots at Bellflower, Kern Medical Center, and Baldwin Park. One of our Bellflower patients came through on a bike — inspired by one of our Thrive commercials. He bought the bike after seeing the commercial.

Colorado has had huge success with drive-thru immunizations — giving more than 100,000 shots to people in cars.

Mid-Atlantic started doing drive-thru's in 2005 — and did 2,700 shots on their first day of "shooting" this year.

Several sites reported giving quite a few shots to people who came by in wheelchairs. Who would have guessed that would happen?

It's a cool thing for us to do. Members like the convenience. Quite a few members say they wouldn't get their shots otherwise.

An unexpected advantage for members is that they don't need to go into a clinic setting full of sick people to get their shots.

One nice thing about being a collaborative organization is that our various sites learn from each other about approaches, promotion strategies, and logistics.

I tend to get my own flu shot in our Oakland office, but I have the advantage of working for a caregiving organization that can make in-office shots available.

Most other folks journey to a medical center of some kind to get their shots. Then after driving to the shot site, they have to park, go into a building, and then usually stand in line to get the needle. It's a lot more convenient to get the shot in the car. Or wheelchair. Or bike.

Drive-by flu shots.

Nice.

Be well.

George

* * *

Background Note: A Good and Full Prevention Agenda Extends to Domestic Violence

We prevent heart attacks, strokes, diabetes, broken bones, premature births and the flu. Some of those programs are highly visible to everyone. We also work hard in a less visible way to prevent domestic violence.

Domestic violence can ruin lives. People don't like to talk about this topic but it is very real. We estimate that over 12,000 of our members will be victims of domestic violence every single month this year. At Kaiser Permanente, we believe we have a dual role — to treat the victims and to help prevent future violence.

The next letter explains some things that we are doing to achieve both of those goals.

Celebrating Our Domestic Violence Prevention Program – October 9, 2009

Dear KP Colleagues,

This week's letter is about a sad and painful topic.

One in four women and one in nine men will experience physical domestic violence in their lifetime. Within our Kaiser Permanente membership, we can estimate that approximately 12,500 people will be the victims of domestic violence every month.

Victims of domestic violence far too often don't get the care they need — often because people who need that care don't know it exists, or because people who need that care are afraid to ask for it.

So why would that topic fit into a weekly celebration letter? We are far from perfect in our programs to help people deal with those sad issues — but we are working hard to do a good job, and our work is being recognized.

We just won a national award for our work.

The people who gave us the award said, "Kaiser Permanente has done extraordinary and truly groundbreaking work to identify and help victims of domestic violence. They have put in place one of the nation's most comprehensive and effective health system responses to domestic violence. As a result, victims in the Kaiser Permanente system are much more likely to get the support and services they need to protect themselves and their children. Kaiser Permanente is truly a model for the country — and the world — in the way it treats victims of domestic violence."

So, Kaiser Permanente has a nationally recognized program for domestic violence prevention and treatment services. The program's coordinated approach includes creating a supportive environment, providing screening and referrals by clinicians, offering onsite domestic violence services, and creating links to appropriate community services.

The program is enhanced by Kaiser Permanente HealthConnect®, our electronic medical record. Our electronic data enables appropriate caregivers to have access to care information that helps us care for all of our patients. KP HealthConnect, includes tools that make it easier for physicians and other caregivers to identify victims of domestic violence, provide a consistent and caring response based on clinical practice recommendations, and make referrals as appropriate to other Kaiser Permanente services and community resources.

This is another case where we learned from ourselves. We are a pioneer in this area.

The Family Violence Prevention Program started as a pilot in one medical facility in Northern California in 1998. It is now being adopted throughout our eight regions. In the Northern California region, with the full set of tools in place, Kaiser Permanente has seen a five-fold increase in the identification of patients dealing with domestic violence.

Domestic violence is a very serious issue. It's an area where people feel great pain and can have their physical wellbeing and their emotional wellbeing damaged and even impaired. We owe it to our members to help where we can and help well.

We are learning as we go. We put a great program in place — and now we are sharing that learning across our system.

You can learn more about our Family Violence Prevention Programs online.

So what I am celebrating this week is a well designed, patient-focused program that helps to improve the quality of life for many of our members, and that caused the Family Violence Prevention Fund to give us their top award.

This is a very good week to celebrate that particular success because October is Domestic Violence Awareness month.

Domestic violence is a sad fact of life. Doing something about it is the right thing to do. Continuously improving our process is an even better thing to do.

So congratulations to our caregivers who make a difference in so many lives.

Be well.

George

* * *

Background Note: We Give Ourselves Awards at Kaiser Permanente for Quality, Safety, Community Service, and Innovation

We like to recognize and celebrate success.

We have set up a whole series of awards programs to do just that inside Kaiser Permanente. We are recognizing and rewarding the behaviors and performance levels that are needed for us to be all that we can be in several key areas.

We love innovation and progress.

We are constantly inventing new ways and improving old ways of delivering care. We have a lovely set of opportunities as a complete care system delivering full care to 9 million people to figure out new and better ways of making care better, safer, more accessible, and more effective.

We like to recognize the people and teams inside Kaiser Permanente who do that work. We believe that giving formal awards can be a very good mechanism for both collective learning and sharing our successes. Quite a few people inside Kaiser Permanente have a good time competing for those awards.

We give four sets of awards every year to our staff and our team. One award is for patient safety. One award is for quality of care. One is for community service. And the fourth award is for innovation.

I usually write one letter each year about each of those awards. So four of my weekly letters each year have been really easy to write — celebrating us recognizing us for doing really good things for us and then sharing what we have learned with us. It's a very "us"-focused process that really helps us create better approaches and better care.

I will not include all of those recognition program letters in this book — but I thought that including a couple of them would give a reader of this book a good sense of what our awards look like and some sense of the kinds of things that our awards recognize.

This next celebration letter is from our KP innovation awards. This letter teed up our most recent annual innovation retreat.

Celebrating Our Innovators Who Are Finding New Ways to Improve Care – April 27, 2012

Dear KP Colleagues,

We are going to celebrate some fun innovation projects next week.

We will be holding our fifth annual Innovation retreat — presenting and recognizing a dozen innovative ways that we are learning to improve care.

Some of the projects are already very ready for prime time. Others are works in progress — with further testing and learning needed before they "go live."

All of them are innovative, and they are all creative in important ways.

One of the in-place projects that will be celebrated next week currently creates a real-time dashboard of hospital capacity at our Northern California hospitals. That project allows us to keep track of every unit's real-time census, and it shows current bed capacity for each site in the entire region from one screen. It's a lovely system.

Another extremely useful project was originally designed to send real-time lab and X-ray results to emergency department clinicians' mobile devices. They now have expanded the project beyond emergency room physicians, and that data can now be accessed by mobile devices of clinicians across the continuum of care. That project is in testing mode. It is very promising.

Another exciting innovation that is being tested involves using new sensors for increased accuracy, and decreasing the time required for X-rays during neurosurgery.

We also implemented a real-time operation support tool at our Northwest primary care clinics. This innovative tool provides operation performance at any level of the organization. It helps the region more proactively manage operations in our clinics. It also helps them more proactively manage access of office visits, patient calls and emails, patient wait times, and actual ED utilization in the moment. The operational intelligence used for this tool is based on a "rules engine" that helps us provide better, more efficient and customized care and service for patients.

Another new project created a prototype of "chat" functionality between members and advice nurses. The world around us is now "chatting." We are learning to do it to improve care.

We also tested technologies that improve infection prevention, enhance interactive patient care, and improve fall-with-injury prevention.

We developed a very elegant prototype for online informed consent for patients, and we prototyped patient decision-making approaches that are aided by viewing online prenatal diagnosis education.

One of the more ambitious projects has created a data model to analyze the impact of room design on patient outcomes and to potentially support real-time decision-making to improve care delivery. This project team took a big-data approach, analyzing more than half a million patient stays in 7,000 patient rooms, to measure the impact of room design on patient outcome.

Another very useful project developed a Web-based tracking application for specimen handoffs. That prototype system improves care by ensuring timely and dependable delivery of specimens to the laboratory.

A very sweet and also useful prototype transmits needed Kaiser Permanente HealthConnect® data from ambulances during patient transport. Again — that can be very important work for some of our patients, because the hospital is more prepared for new arrivals.

We are doing an amazing number of innovative things. Patient care is our focus — and we are inventing, building, and testing truly innovative new tools to make care better.

It will be a fun Innovation retreat to attend.

So my letter this week celebrates our innovators — the really creative people who are figuring out how to make care better in big ways and small … and I am also celebrating and thanking the development teams and the actual caregivers who are making those creative ideas real and useful.

Great stuff.

Well done.

Be well.

George

* * *

Background Note: The Quality Award Nominees Get Better Every Year

The annual quality award weekly letter is also a really fun letter to write. We have a lot of quality improvement agendas at Kaiser Permanente. The impact of those agendas is very basic. The national measurement of health care quality in the country comes from the NCQA (National Committee for Quality Assurance). NCQA provides the HEDIS (Healthcare Effectiveness Data and Information Set) quality care report. More than 1,000 plans are measured by the HEDIS process. Quite a few lists of HEDIS scores have the top score in the country with Kaiser Permanente as the very best plan.

Those quality successes are not accidental. They also don't happen in a static environment. Continuous improvement is a continuous process. It is also a comprehensive process. This year's weekly letter about our internal quality award winner also celebrated the other 14 quality award nominees for the Vohs Quality Award inside Kaiser Permanente. We have some very bright people doing some really good work in a lot of settings.

It is always really hard work every year for the quality award selection committee to pick just one winner from all of the nominated programs.

Celebrating the 2012 20th Annual James A. Vohs Award for Quality – March 23, 2012

Dear KP Colleagues,

Winning the James A. Vohs Award for Quality is not easy at Kaiser Permanente because the competition is so fierce.

We just had 15 nominees for the annual James A. Vohs Award for Quality. Fifteen great internal Kaiser Permanente quality programs were nominated for the award.

One of the programs that was nominated significantly reduced the 30-day mortality and morbidity levels for surgical patients — including developing and implementing an improved pneumonia prevention protocol.

Another program significantly improved care follow-up for osteo-arthritis patients using shared decision making and improved care intervention.

Another program focused on improving the patient education process for diabetic patients — enhancing educational levels and improving nutritional management for patients.

Another nominee for the Vohs Award improved patient screening by linking radiology resources to other patient visits and worked out successful scripts to be used in calling overdue patients to encourage them to get their mammograms.

Another program focused on hospital-acquired infections for kids — with an emphasis on neonatal intensive care patients, ventilator-associated pneumonias, and bloodstream infections related to central lines for kids.

That program has been a huge success — almost eliminating ventilator-assisted pneumonias (VAP) infections for kids for the last couple of years. The learnings from that program and that hospital are being shared across all KP hospitals with those patients.

Another nominated program was set up to do improved screening for chest pain in patients. The goal was to identify more accurately which patients needed hospitalization. The screening plan also included an integrated and focused discharge plan that included better and clearer patient education about both cardiovascular risk and appropriate preventive therapies. That program significantly improved the accuracy level for admissions.

One of the most interesting nominees for the Vohs Award focused on physician training and enculturation. To help new physicians move more quickly to full effectiveness as members of the KP care team, our Orange County service area created a special onboarding program based on "Schein's Theory of Organizational Socialization (OS)."

The sponsors of the program said that the effort was worthy of consideration as a Vohs Award for Quality winner because patients are safer faster when the new doctors come fully up to speed very quickly on our processes and our approaches.

Another nominee for the award also made the point that great training is very useful. The Surgical Care Information Project set up a checklist and a well-designed process for best practices for surgical care. That program includes training as well as post-operative follow-up tracking mechanisms for patients and doctors.

We had another nominated project reduce the rate of central line-associated bloodstream infections by 65 percent over a two-year period by implementing the Comprehensive Unit-Based Safety Program (CUSP). Some of the program's strategies that made it so successful involved formation of a CUSP Team, development of a safety culture, and physician engagement.

Another one of the nominated projects — in efforts to improve glycemic control practices — launched a program which implemented as a core program component a Glycemic Control Pharmacy Team to increase glycemic control in perioperative patients by providing expert glycemic management in the perioperative period.

That special team proved to be the strongest of the program's many components that served to reduce all cause readmission rates from 15.2 to 8.1 percent and reduced 90-day emergency room visits from 24.1 to 15.2 percent.

And yet another nominated program also addressing glycemic levels involved intensive glycemic monitoring of women with gestational diabetes. Their glucose levels were monitored four times a day rather than the usual once every two weeks. That new strategy resulted in an overall 33 percent decrease in the number of C-sections performed on patients with gestational diabetes.

Those programs have all improved care. Each of those nominated programs is an asset to patients and to KP as a care system.

In addition to those excellent programs, four other nominees were awarded finalist status by the Vohs Award Evaluation Committee.

One of the four Vohs Award finalists was a lovely program set up in Southern California to significantly increase the number of chronic care patients who are taking their medications.

Southern California created a "Medication Adherence Tool" that triggers a report on each patient that can be used by our physicians, nurse practitioners, physician assistants, case managers, panel managers, and our clinical pharmacists to identify patients who are not refilling their prescriptions.

That approach used direct phone calls, letters, and automated calls, and then added the information to the "Care Everywhere" support system.

How well did it work?

We ended up with a 62 percent better refill rate with the new program. That result will obviously make care outcomes better for a lot of people.

Another lovely Southern California program that was also a Vohs Award finalist was our Heart Failure Transitional Care Program.

The heart failure program used a team of caregivers to design a regionally standardized system to guide care through safe transitions from hospital to home.

That heart patient transitions program has created a seamless level of care for our high-risk heart failure patients. The program decreased the readmission rate for those patients by 30 percent and — more importantly — it saved an estimated 410 lives.

Four hundred lives are a lot of lives to save. Four hundred families were spared the tragedy of a death because that program did its job and did it well.

The third Vohs Award for Quality finalist also comes from Southern California. The Orthopedic Total Joint Replacement Pain Protocol performance team focused on improving patient safety by eliminating adverse drug reactions relative to pain medications.

The program also optimized pain management for Kaiser Permanente patients following total joint replacements.

The program used a collaborative multidisciplinary system that did that work, and that team set a goal of no SRAEs (Serious Reportable Adverse Events) in addition to improving the pain levels for the patients whose joints were replaced.

Again — patients' lives and care outcomes were better because very bright and deeply concerned caregivers figured out a better set of processes for the care of those patients.

Great people did great work and made a difference in a lot of lives.

So with all of those really impressive and successful programs as nominees, what program did the Vohs Award Committee select for the official Vohs winner for 2012?

The Vohs Award went to another lovely program that made great use of our computer database to identify patients at risk for kidney disease.

That program set up uniquely proactive consultations and team care for our nephrologists and primary care patients in Hawaii. Hawaii is the perfect place to make a real difference in kidney care because the native Hawaiian population has particularly high level of risk for kidney disease.

The program was entirely proactive — sorting through our computerized care data to identify patients at high risk of kidney failure and then getting those patients specific intervention plans with primary care doctors and nephrologists working as a team to help patients protect and preserve their kidneys. The intervention process improved the early referrals to nephrology from 53 to 89 percent of patients reaching end stage renal disease.

Early interventions significantly improve the success levels. The relative risk of progression was reduced by 46 percent from Stage 3A to 3B, and by 40 percent from Stage 3 to Stage 4/5.

Those are a lot of numbers. It also represents a lot of people.

Each of those numbers represents real people who did not have their personal health status deteriorate to Stage 4/5 kidney failure status. Stage 4/5 status is really not a good place to be.

So the Hawaii program saved lives, improved lives, and made great use of our database and our team approach to care to truly improve care.

Our nephrology and primary care approach in Hawaii was the winner of the Vohs Award in 2012. It was the first Vohs Award win for the Hawaii Region.

Hawaii has had a number of other quality wins — including achieving first place scores for the entire country on some National Committee for Quality Assurance/Healthcare Effectiveness Data and Information Set (NCQA/HEDIS) quality measures, but this was the first Vohs win.

So my letter this week celebrates the Vohs winner and finalists. I am also celebrating all of the 15 great programs that were nominated for the Vohs Award for Quality.

But the real winners are our patients. Care is better for our patients because the caregivers of Kaiser Permanente are doing great work in so many areas.

We have a lot of care improvement programs going on at Kaiser Permanente. No care system is perfect. But we can strive to be great, and we can work hard to get continuously better.

The Vohs Award recognized that we are on that trail again.

Well done, care teams.

Be well.

George

✳ ✳ ✳

Background Note: The Patient Safety Award Nominees Get Better Every Year As Well

Patient safety is extremely important to us. Across the country, we know that millions of patients end up suffering from adverse negative care experiences as the result of infections, mistakes, and errors.

We are focused as a care system on being continuously better in all of these areas. As part of that focus, we give annual internal awards for patient safety, as well.

The last couple of letters celebrated our quality improvement awards and our innovation awards. We also are doing some very good work on patient safety — and our most recent patient safety awards dinner gave me the choice to write another very easy-to-write celebration letter.

Patients need safe care. We know for an absolute fact that safe care does not happen by accident. We also know that good intentions are not enough to create safety. A lot of very well intentioned care sites in this country are not very safe.

Safe care needs to be built and designed and implemented. Safe practices need to be implemented and then fiercely protected. Why protected? Safety programs need to be guarded and protected over time by people who really want care to be continuously safe because the sad truth is that care can default very quickly to unsafe levels. That default can happen very quickly — as soon as any organization or care site stops paying attention to safety. Care is not naturally safe. Safety is a never-ending agenda and function.

But safety is possible. Safe care can happen.

The next letter about this year's patient safety awards makes that point.

Celebrating the 2011 David Lawrence Patient Safety Awards – January 6, 2012

Dear KP Colleagues,

One program cut the number of pressure ulcers in a hospital to zero for nearly a year.

Another program cut the number of medication errors by more than half.

Another program helped high risk patients in times of transitions from care site to care site.

Another program reduced the increase, abuse, and risk of OxyContin use.

Yet another program created rapid-response teams that achieved a 47 percent reduction in patients needing "code" level of care.

Another program set up extensive training programs using mannequins and computerized patients to improve team care and patient response techniques and approaches.

Another program decreased therapeutic misuse of acetaminophen.

What do all of those programs have in common?

They are all Kaiser Permanente programs that have been nominated for the David Lawrence Patient Safety Award. They are all programs we have created at Kaiser Permanente to better the care of our patients.

We have done some very good work on patient safety.

We care deeply about the safety of our patients — and we know and believe that patient safety happens because we, as a care team, do the right things to keep patients safe.

It's a learning experience. It's also a process of continuous improvement. We put processes and programs in place to make care better and safer. We learn from others and we learn from ourselves.

Some great safety programs have been developed and implemented by us. The programs listed above were among dozens of programs that were invented by Kaiser Permanente care sites and nominated for the annual David Lawrence Patient Safety Award.

So who won this year's awards?

We actually give two awards every year — one award for a brand-new safety project and one award to the region and care team who did the best job of transferring and implementing the work of a prior winner. We are often our own best teachers and our own best students. The David Lawrence Patient Safety Award for a New Project was awarded this year to the Northwest Region for its "Transition Care" program.

Transition care is extremely important — because we want our patients who transition from our care sites back to their homes to have the best possible recovery from the treatments. Doing a great job of supporting that transition takes clear thinking, effective processes, systematic approaches, and dedicated caregivers who help patients make those transfers.

That was the new project winner.

The Lawrence Patient Safety Transfer Award for successfully implementing a prior year's winning submission to a new region went to the Colorado Region for its successful implementation of a specimen-handling program that won the Lawrence Award a year ago for the Anatomical Specimen Handling Reliability Project.

The Lawrence Patient Safety Award Selection Committee also honored the Northern California Region this year for its "Automated Patient Safety Threat Detection & Feedback" program. That program very nicely uses Kaiser Permanente HealthConnect® for quality and risk monitoring. That risk detection project very skillfully incorporates the Institute for Healthcare Improvement's "Global Trigger Tool" to identify potential threats to patients in real time.

The Colorado Region had a very good year on safety awards and was also recognized for its "Drug Renal Intervention Program." That program reduces medical errors caused by dispensing inappropriate doses or medications to patients with renal disease.

Safety matters.

Safety saves lives.

Safety is not an accident and it doesn't happen just because good people are well intentioned and try hard.

Safety is a thought process and a skill set and it is a commitment by caring people to do smart and safe things for our patients.

We are continuously improving our safety agenda.

THE PATIENT SAFETY AWARD NOMINEES GET BETTER EVERY YEAR AS WELL

My letter this week celebrates the Kaiser Permanente patient safety programs that were so distinctive and well done that they earned Lawrence Award recognition.

Well done.

George

☆ ☆ ☆

Background Note: We Earn Outside Awards As Well – Outside Recognition Programs Tend To Rate Us Highly

Health care performance levels used to be totally invisible. Years ago, no one really knew at any level how well any care site, care team, or health plan compared in performance relative to any other care site, care team or health plan.

Ignorance was not bliss. Bad performance happened a lot, and it was almost always invisible. In that date-free world, care did not continuously improve. The bad performers too often did not improve because the truth is that most bad care sites are well intentioned, and those poorly performing care sites usually believe strongly that they were doing great work when no data existed. Bad performers in many sites believed their care to be good until someone showed them actual data on their problematic performance. That problem of invisible performance is now getting at least partially resolved.

There are a growing number of very important external programs that now rate many levels of health care delivery and health plan performance.

We love those programs. We learn from those comparative databases. They help guide our thinking. It is very good to know when we are doing well, and it is vital and extremely important to know when we are not.

We generally tend to do very well in those external recognitions of service, quality, and performance. We have won recognitions for our diversity, quality of care, service levels, status as a place to work, and our safety levels. We have won awards for being green — environmentally responsible — and we have won awards for being good citizens.

The next letter describes an award we won for having the very best lab in America. We were rated the number one medical laboratory for the country.

The letter is a little longer than most of my letters because I wanted all of our people to see the kinds of specific activities, achievements, processes, data gathering, and performance levels that were needed for us to win the best lab in the country award.

Celebrating Laboratory of the Year – May 11, 2012

Dear KP Colleagues,

The Medical Laboratory Observer (MLO) is a nationally recognized, peer-reviewed management journal for laboratory professionals.

Every year, the MLO looks across all of the hospital and clinical laboratories in the United States, and they select one laboratory to be the National Laboratory of the Year.

They rate laboratories based on service levels, performance, and on each lab's focus on patients.

They also rate laboratories based on their "commitment to laboratory science, to professionalism, to teamwork, and most of all — to serving the public health."

So how did we do in that national rating of laboratories?

We won.

Our Panorama City Medical Center Laboratory was just named Laboratory of the Year ☑ for the entire country.

There were two runners up — a laboratory in Missouri and a laboratory in Oregon.

We were ranked number one.

It's very good to be great at being a laboratory.

Our laboratories are incredibly important to us. Our patients need their laboratory tests done quickly and well. We spend a lot of time and resources putting in place the equipment and facilities and the processes needed to meet our patients' laboratory test needs.

"Needs" is the right word.

Our patients need our labs.

So do our caregivers.

More than two-thirds of all medical decisions are informed by laboratory tests of one kind or another.

So how are we doing with our laboratories?

Our service levels are now setting the standard for health care.

As I mentioned in an earlier letter, I had my blood drawn on the way to work one day last month. One of our laboratories processed the blood that morning.

I personally had the results of the tests on my iPhone by 11 that same morning.

That is a lovely level of functionality.

In almost any other care setting, that kind of rapid response would be "concierge" care — special care done for very few patients for a very high additional price.

We do it for nine million patients all the time.

Literally all the time.

Continuously.

We actually average 81,000 laboratory results every day that are viewed electronically by our patients.

More than 100 laboratory results have been sent out electronically to patients in the time it took anyone to read the first part of this letter.

Overall — across all of our care sites, hospitals and clinics — we now run and use 150 million laboratory tests a year.

Those are both big numbers and real people.

Every one of those laboratory tests involves a patient and a process — and millions of care decisions result from all of that information.

The lives of people are affected hugely by those tests.

So it is a really good thing for us to be good at doing laboratory tests.

And it is very reinforcing when a leading journal in the laboratory management industry believes our performance is good enough to rate us as the very best.

So why and how did our Panorama City Medical Center Laboratory achieve the top award? The MLO mentioned several factors in the award announcement. They pointed out that —

89 percent of our surveyed patients indicated that they are "definitely satisfied" with the lab's overall service. The laboratory had 83 percent of patients who reported having waited less than five minutes for service.

The laboratory achieved the lowest percentage of member complaints — with a really well done, very low 0.02 percent of members complaining, out of a total of more than 300,000 laboratory outpatient interactions.

Prioritizing patient care — our Kaiser Permanente laboratory achieved phenomenal results by prioritizing a series of commitments to patient care. Zero labeling error was achieved by the implementation of a wireless handheld positive patient ID system. Zero is a great number.

The laboratory also actively participated in the care teams' Stroke Accreditation Committee, and has consistently achieved a turnaround time of less than 45 minutes for code stroke patients.

The laboratory's critical result documentation was 99.7 percent in compliance. Its blood culture contamination rate of 1.62 percent, including both phlebotomist and nurse draws — and representing more than 18,000 cultures — was below the national contamination average of three percent by nearly one-half.

Team care is a major reason for our success. The team in that lab meets monthly to discuss laboratory issues and come up with workflow improvements and solutions. Among the improvements were:

A working "TAT" Dashboard. The turnaround time dashboard monitored turnaround times for CLS and laboratory assistants resulted in the Panorama City laboratory having the best ER turnaround time in the region.

A color-coded system to quickly differentiate samples coming from the ER, surgery, and stroke patients. The implementation of this elegant and lovely system significantly improved the turnaround times for code stroke and surgical patients. The system allows prioritization and quick reporting of results when both precision and speed are needed most to save patients' lives.

Coordinated with the Regional Reference Laboratory, staff worked to reduce specimen rejections. That work led to Panorama City having the lowest send-out rejection rate in the region — 0.1 percent.

Maximizing productivity and quality control: Every month, each laboratory manager/supervisor, along with a staff member, performs four to six observations to ensure workplace safety. Out of the total of 120 employees, Panorama City had only two incidents of on-the-job injury in 2011, for a total of just three work days lost. Not one single needlestick accident was reported for the entire year. Again — zero is a great number. The Unit Based Team focus on that issue helped the lab become the number one laboratory in the region for workplace safety in 2011.

The laboratory also participated in inter-laboratory quality control programs for BioRad Chemistry and Beckman Coulter hematology. The laboratory achieved 99 percent accuracy on proficiency testing for regulated analytes.

Continuing education is also a reason for the laboratory being rated number one in the country. Panorama City does a great job of keeping everyone current.

We also do a significant amount of community service with the lab. The Kaiser Permanente Mobile Health Vehicle is set up frequently at previously announced locations in the communities around us.

Those are the reasons why our Panorama City laboratory was just recognized as being the best laboratory in the entire country.

That really is a lovely and well deserved recognition.

So my letter this week celebrates our entire laboratory team — all of the people at Kaiser Permanente who do all of those tests and do them with a very high degree of accuracy and a high level of performance and a real focus on service.

Great work, KP laboratory teams.

And my letter also celebrates the lab team at Panorama City.

Laboratory of the Year.

Well done.

Be well.

George

✳ ✳ ✳

Background Note: Making the Right Thing Easy to Do^(SM)

Making the right thing easy to do is our mantra.

Our approach at Kaiser Permanente is to think hard about how we can systematically make things better. We have systems, solutions, and systems improvement approaches as a primary problem-solving approach. A problem-solving work or care environment that focuses only on each specific problem as an individual crisis and as a separate incident may solve the incident — but there is a high likelihood that the negative incident will occur and reoccur, and then the problem will have to be solved over and over again — maybe every single day in many care settings.

We hate that incident-centered approach. We would much rather figure out ways of changing the process of care delivery to fix each major problem once and have it stay fixed. Rather than put the wrong hip into patients and then have to redo the surgery over and over again, we would rather figure out what implant is the best and what surgical approach is best and then redo the hip surgery half as many times because we did it right the first time.

One of our most important internal intellectual and strategic guide posts is to "Make The Right Thing Easy To Do." Those are powerful words. We set that very specific guideline and thought process as an operational goal for almost everything we do. It is an elegant, lovely, clear, functional and highly useful context for looking at all of our functions and goals.

"Making the right thing easy to do" is a mantra for our systems design teams. It is the focusing mission for the people in our Care Management Institute (CMI) — a group of brilliant people who work every day to keep our Kaiser Permanente care team current and well-supported with Medical Best Practices.

The next celebration letter deals with that mantra and that agenda. The letter explains why sending pharmacy refills by mail to patients' homes increases compliance levels and improves care outcomes for patients, because taking the medication is clearly the "Right Thing To Do." And so we decided to "Make It Easy" with our processes and our approaches to getting prescriptions filled.

"Make the right thing easy to do." That deceptively simple guideline has an elegance, a functionality, and a power that has to be experienced in the real world to be believed.

Celebrating Making the Right Thing Easy to Do – August 12, 2011

Dear KP Colleagues,

The basic goal, philosophy, agenda, role, and motto of the Kaiser Permanente Care Management Institute (CMI) has been — for over fourteen years — to "Make The Right Thing Easy To Do."

That sounds like a simple mission. At one level, it is.

At another level, it is an incredible, elegant, insightful, and quintessentially functional reason for CMI to exist.

That CMI motto doesn't just apply to CMI. It applies to our whole organization. Making the right thing easy to do improves both health and care in a wide range of areas.

When I talk to outside audiences about us making the right thing easy to do, I always point out that the process inherently comes with two separate and very important parts. Part one: Figure out the right thing. Part two: Make it easy to do.

Each of those agendas is individually important. For any given patient, situation, disease, or issue, figuring out the right thing is obviously extremely important.

We have very smart people who spend time and energy figuring out a lot of right things to do.

Then the challenge is to figure out how to make that right thing easy to do.

What does that double process look like in the real world? Taking care of chronic care patients is one example.

We are particularly good at providing team care to our patients with chronic conditions. One element of right care is right medications. We know what the right medications are for each patient.

We also know that most of our chronic care patients should take their medications daily, usually forever.

That is a right thing.

Once we figure out the right medication for each patient, we then need to figure out how we can help make taking that medication by the patient easy to do.

Owning pharmacies helps. It is very convenient for the patient when we have our own pharmacy in the same building with the patient's physicians. Having pharmacies in close proximity to the physician's office obviously helps make the right thing easy to do for patients who are in that office after they get the prescriptions.

We may have the highest success level in the country for having patients actually pick up their initial medications.

Best, however, wasn't good enough. We also wanted to increase the percentage of chronic care patients who both fill and refill their prescriptions.

Multiple studies show very low compliance levels across the country for American patients refilling their prescriptions.

What could we do to improve our refill success levels?

We know that even when the pharmacy is in the same building as the patient's physician, getting refills on prescriptions almost always involves travel time for patients.

Travel time for patients can make the right thing to do, hard to do. Travel can be inconvenient — not easy.

We weren't happy with the number of patients who didn't come in to do their prescription renewals.

So what did we do?

We eliminated the need for most patients to come in to pick up refills.

We started mailing prescriptions to the patients.

That definitely made the right thing easy to do for many patients. It's definitely easier to open your mailbox than it is to drive to the clinic.

So how well did that strategy work?

We did a study.

Our research team in Northern California did a study to see if more chronic care patients refilled their prescriptions if mail order pharmacy was an option.

The study, done by our Division of Research, is called "The Comparative Effectiveness of Mail Order Pharmacy Use vs. Local Pharmacy Use on LDL-C Control in New Statin Users."

Getting prescriptions for patients by mail worked.

Our researchers found that 84.7 percent of patients who received their medications by mail at least two-thirds of the time stuck to their physician-prescribed regimen, versus 76.9 percent who picked up their medications at "brick and mortar" Kaiser Permanente pharmacies.

Higher levels of prescription refill success for chronic care drugs will result in fewer heart attacks, fewer kidney failures, and a reduction in other chronic care related crises.

More than two hundred news outlets wrote or told stories last week about the study.

Other care teams now know that refill success can be improved with mail order pharmacy delivery.

It's a good and smart thing to do. We made the right thing easy to do, and more people did the right thing.

You can see one of the articles written about our care improvement success here.

So that is a key strategy for us.

Make the right thing easy to do.

My letter this week celebrates both the folks who figured out the right thing and the folks who made it easy to do.

Well done.

Be well.
George

* * *

Background Note: We Want the Best and Most Current Medical Knowledge and Science Available to Our Caregivers in Real Time

We very much want our caregivers to have constant access to the best medical knowledge and science.

The science of medicine changes regularly. We want all of our caregivers to have efficient and convenient access to medical journals, medical research, medical information updates, and medical protocols.

We also want to make that process of getting access to medical knowledge "Easy to Do." This is our mantra. It's always good when we can "Make The Right Thing Easy To Do."

So we have created a user-friendly electronic medical library.

Our electronic medical library is incredibly important work.

We make the right thing easy to do by giving our caregivers great and convenient access to the best medical science and to the best care protocols. There are huge numbers of medical journals being published daily. Medical science evolves all of the time.

It is extremely hard — if not impossible — for any single, solo caregiver anywhere to keep up with the explosion of medical information.

We want our caregivers to "keep up" — so we have implemented an electronic medical library to make keeping up easy to do.

That library gets constant use — as you can read in the next celebration letter. Our electronic medical library definitely "Makes The Right Thing Easy To Do." Very few care sites in America have a tool that does this kind of work. That is a shame. Every caregiver in America should have access to an equivalent medical library — as you will see when you read the next letter.

Celebrating Our New Computerized Clinical Library – February 11, 2011

Dear KP Colleagues,

Everyone knows that we have the most complete and largest civilian electronic medical record in the world. People also know that our care-givers now have made great progress towards our goal of having "all of the information, about all of our patients, all of the time" as part of KP HealthConnect® data system.

What people don't know is that we also have one of the largest, most complete and most inclusive electronic medical information libraries in the world. Our electronic medical library has current and easy-to-access information about care, care delivery, best practices, and pure medical science in easy-to-use and easy-to-access formats.

We have built a lovely care support tool to help us be a learning organization and a learning care team.

Our new electronic care library is a great new tool for our caregivers. The tool is getting used.

On an average day, there are more than 10,000 uses of our computerized medical library by our medical care team. The system is used by our 15,000 physicians and it is used by other KP caregivers who need clinical information. We had slightly over 82,000 unique clinical visitors in January alone. The information is there when needed — and it is even available in the exam room at the point of care.

Those 10,000 daily uses happen because that data site is one of the largest and easiest to use computerized clinical libraries. Our Clinical Library website is run by our Care Management Institute (CMI) and it contains data from thousands of medical sources.

Data includes medical science, recommended best practices, proven care protocols, and — to make our physicians' practice lives easier — it contains links and advice for the physicians to use to order services and arrange for tests and procedures from our total KP staff and care system.

The goal is to make access to that information easy.

The basic philosophy of the Care Management Institute is exactly that — to "make the right thing easy to do."

"Make the right thing easy to do" is actually an incredibly profound guideline. Why? Making the right thing easy to do hugely increases the likelihood that the right thing will be done.

That CMI philosophy has two parts — 1) figuring out the right thing and then 2) making it easy to do.

Many electronic medical record systems in other care sites have been unsuccessful or some have even failed because the people putting the systems together were not focused on making the right thing easy to do.

Caregivers in non-Kaiser Permanente care sites and settings often have to wrestle with paper databases for their medical science information and don't have access to any research or best practice data in real time or even on a delayed basis in the actual exam room. Our new on-site comprehensive functionality simply does not exist in other care environments... and that makes delivering care in those other care settings both harder and less well informed in many cases. Those other care sites are often not set up to make the right thing easy to do.

Our KP Care Management Institute was founded many years ago to accomplish that lovely dual mission — figuring out the right thing and then making it easy to do.

Our new web portal for care information does exactly that set of work. The electronic library has great resources about medical science, and it is set up to make using those resources easier to access and use.

We have been getting better at creating this level of access every year.

The new system is 40 percent more accessible than the old system — measured by how long it took to find specific information in the old computer library for medical care topics compared to the time it takes today to find the same information.

So what is in the electronic libraries?

We have guidelines and member handouts that are region specific. We have 1,500 online journals and several hundred textbooks. We have ways to get continuing education, member class schedules, and colleague phone numbers. We have information that has general across-the-board usefulness, and information that can be used to calculate basic data for individual patients.

The new system allows for more efficient content maintenance. It is set up to do instantaneous revisions when old data needs to be improved and replaced. In other care sites outside of Kaiser Permanente, it can take months or even years to get an important new piece of medical information to caregivers. We can do it in minutes.

The system allows for both faster and less expensive dissemination of best practices and new medical information across Kaiser Permanente.

It is an effective tool to use. It offers a single site for all clinical content, so people don't need to hunt for information in separate systems set up for each medical specialty. The information is categorized but it is not siloed.

We created this new system on a foundation of earlier electronic library support systems.

The legacy systems all had their usefulness and charm. Colorado joined an early version of a national computerized medical library system back in 2003. Northern California and Northwest moved their own electronic libraries to that same early national system while Mid-Atlantic and Hawaii built their own regional systems on the computer and the web in 2004. Southern California went live with computerized medical library services in 2005, and Georgia went live with a computerized medical library in 2009.

Each of the prior systems was studied to examine the questions that were asked and the support services that were needed. The new system reflects that work and that learning process.

Now we have a complete combined system that builds on all of those foundational legacy systems, provides a wider scope of information, and is designed for easier and more convenient use.

The new system became operational last month.

So my letter this week celebrates all the folks at CMI and in all of the regions who have built a highly efficient, easy-to-use, functionally integrated electronic medical science and best practice library and database and made it operational for all of our caregivers.

CMI — Making the right thing easy to do.

That library — all by itself — is an incredibly powerful, effective, right thing to do.

Be well.

George

* * *

Background Note: We Want to Bake Innovation Into Our Approach to Care

We are a fairly large caregiving organization. We actually have the largest private medical groups in the world. We are one of the largest hospital systems in the country. We probably are the largest in-house private pharmacy system in the world, and we are definitely one of the largest imaging caregivers in the world. There are very few laboratory systems anywhere bigger than ours.

We deliver a lot of care and we deliver most of that care on sites that we directly own. That means that we have had to learn to be very good at designing, building, reengineering, and using sites of care.

Care is evolving every day. We not only need to be good at yesterday's care and today's care, we need to be good at tomorrow's care.

To help with that process, we have built a relatively unique innovation center in Northern California that has received recognition around the world for doing some very useful work to improve care delivery.

The next letter celebrates that center.

We named our innovation center the Garfield Innovation Center after our founding physician — Sidney Garfield, M.D. Doctor Garfield was a brilliant innovator. He actually started building electronic medical records decades before anyone else even thought of it. He innovated in multiple ways — so this letter celebrates both Dr. Garfield and the special center we set up in his name.

Celebrating The Garfield Innovation Center – April 4, 2008

Dear KP Colleagues,

Earlier this year, I wrote a weekly letter celebrating our use of robots — mechanical replicas of people — as training tools for our caregivers. We are pioneering that work and it is going really well.

The robots give birth, have strokes, pass out, and give our caregivers great training opportunities.

Two weeks later, I wrote about our computer simulations of patients — our "virtual people" — who dwell in our Archimedes system. I described how the computer simulations of patients were extremely useful in predicting the efficacy of care patterns and the progression of disease in real people.

So with one set of staff using mechanical replicas of people and another set of staff using electronic replicas of people, I suspect it won't surprise anyone to learn that we also create Hollywood-like full scale mockups and physical models of care sites so we can study, design and re-engineer actual care delivery sites — at times using actors who pretend to be our patients.

In our Sidney Garfield Innovation Center just south of Oakland, we have a large warehouse-like building that has inside it an interesting set of fake hospital rooms and fake care delivery sites.

The Garfield Center lets us move walls around, move doorways, move electrical connections, move bed locations, and — in essence — continuously re-engineer the actual physical sites of care without us ever interfering with the flow of care for a real patient.

We do sometimes have real patients visit our care-site mockups at the Garfield Center to give us patient-focused feedback on our various design experiments and ideas.

The Center has over 30,000 square feet of space, and includes a fully furnished medical prep room, an emergency treatment room, a labor and delivery room, nursing stations, patient care rooms, and exam rooms, along with a complete clinic layout where needed.

I mentioned two weeks ago that we have over five thousand active facility-related building, repair, upgrade or expansion projects going on at Kaiser Permanente in 2008. We are investing billions of dollars in care site construction. It would be irresponsible of us not to take competent steps to be sure we are building sites that do their job really well.

In addition to the Hollywood back lot, process re-enactment aspect of the Garfield Center, it is also a place where new technology is test-driven before it is purchased. Nurse medication carts provide a good example of a "successful failure." Nurses tested the carts and found that while they reduced the number of trips back and forth from patient rooms, they created a whole host of other problems including ergonomic difficulties for our staff. Two tests run by the Garfield Center with frontline nurses determined that the carts were good in concept, but a poor solution in reality.

So that's the goal, role, and job of the Garfield Center. Real caregivers play around with — and experiment with — physical simulations of our various care sites.

I've visited the center a couple of times. People on that team seem to be very highly engaged and highly energized.

We have had a number of visitors from all over the world who have walked through that center. It's one of our most popular "show and tell" sites. The fact that we have that center and use it as we do tells all of those visitors that we are serious about being on the "cutting edge" of figuring out and delivering right care.

It is particularly appropriate to name the center after Dr. Sidney Garfield — one of our co-founders. Dr. Garfield and Henry Kaiser worked together to create what has become Kaiser Permanente. Both were inventors. Both were pioneers.

Dr. Garfield was an unquestioned visionary. His statement to the American Medical Association in 1971 about the future value of computers to physicians was an insight of sheer genius.

Some physicians back in 1965 were resisting or even fearing computers. Dr. Garfield gave a speech where he said, "As physicians, you can benefit in many ways. With computerized history and findings available...you will know more about your patients than you do today. You will be able to serve them better and treat them more rationally...Your work will be more interesting and stimulating."

Or as Dr. Garfield told medical students a decade later at the University of Southern California in 1975, "One can envision a new health care system...that...will chart each individual's personal pathway through our health care resources toward optimal health. Periodic updating of health evaluation profiles...will trigger computerized warnings and corrective instructions....Such individualized continuing healthcare would...optimize the health of each individual through his (or her) lifetime. It should be clear this...could never be fully achieved without the large amount of individual information, cybernetic data feedback, protocols, advice rules, monitoring and surveillance that systematized health evaluation and computerization makes possible. Supplementing today's sick care services with this new system in providing the accessibility it makes possible can raise the quality and distribution of U.S. medicine to a level unparalleled in the world. That is the great promise of this new delivery system for medicine of the future."

KP HealthConnect® is very obviously a direct linear extension of that intellectual and perceptional insight and understanding.

So naming our frontline care site innovation center in honor of Dr. Garfield makes perfect sense.

We celebrated our mechanical patients and our electronic simulations of patients in prior weeks. This week I am celebrating the actors who work in the Garfield Center to portray our patients — and I am celebrating the entire Garfield Center team and program for their cutting edge work on site design.

You can see more about the Garfield Center on the KP portal.

Have a great week and be well.

George

* * *

Background Note: We Also Need to Deliver Great Palliative Care

Some patients in the last stages of terminal illnesses need very special, very highly focused care. We need to be there with great skill and great compassion for those patients.

When all other care has lost its ability to help the patient, we really need to be very good at meeting patient needs for palliative care.

So another major area of patient-focused innovation for our Kaiser Permanente care teams has been in the area of palliative care.

We work hard to save lives. We have been consistently successful. We may have the best mortality rates for heart disease, diabetes, and for our HIV patients. Our cancer mortality rates are also better than the U.S. average — in some cases, significantly better. We work hard and well to keep our patients alive. We do better than most care programs in many areas. But we are not always successful. Some patients get to the point where the right care for the patient is palliative care.

When patients are terminal, the right level and type of palliative care can be one of the most important things in their lives. Palliative care is a labor of love, and it takes real commitment and very caring people to help people at the time in their lives when palliative help really is needed.

My next weekly letter celebrated our continuously improving patient-focused approaches to palliative care. This was also one of my very first weekly letters. I mention that it was an early letter because the number of KP hospitals that is mentioned in the letter has expanded since that letter was written. We now have 37 hospitals, with a couple more on the way. We have also now expanded the palliative care teams to all of our care sites. It was the right thing to do.

Celebrating Palliative Care – November 30, 2007

Dear KP Colleagues,

When my uncle was dying in Northern Minnesota, he was absolutely clear that he wanted to die at home in his own bed, cared for by my aunt and his daughters.

He had two choices — to lie in the hospital in a strange room without enough chairs and no place for his wife or daughters to rest or freshen up. Or he could die in his own home, his own bed, supported and surrounded by people he loved and who loved him.

He was blessed to have the option of a palliative care program, an in home hospice which was run by the local hospital. The hospice caregivers helped him with basic support, helped with his medications, some counseling and helped his family understand and anticipate the actual dying process.

When he breathed his last breath, his daughter was sitting by the bed. She knew exactly what had happened and what needed to be done. It was all loving, respectful, considerate, and a very supportive way of dealing with what is inherently a sad and painful process.

Why do I mention that particular experience that happened in Northern Minnesota in one of my weekly celebration letters?

I mention it because we at Kaiser Permanente have been doing some very good work in rolling out our own palliative care program that provides comparable levels of very special care for people in that same time of need. We now have that program in place in all 32 of our own hospitals and in five partner hospitals.

My aunt was extremely grateful for the program that supported my uncle. Helping people with their pain is a very good thing to do. Helping people who are dying with an in-home care support system is a very good thing to do.

Our own Kaiser Permanente program was piloted in Colorado, San Francisco, and Portland. We studied the results. Patient and family satisfaction levels were extremely high. A very bright and caring team of well trained and collaborative caregivers put together processes, approaches, training programs and care protocols that are exceptional, patient-focused, and aimed at providing our patients with the levels of care needed in those challenging times. Patients rate our programs extremely high for quality of care and both emotional and spiritual support of care. Chaplains are involved in many palliative care teams, as well as doctors, nurses and social workers.

Members of our palliative care staff have received formal Education on Palliative and End-of-Life Care (EPEC) or End-of-Life Nursing Education Consortium (ELNEC) training, including symptom control and pain management. Kaiser Permanente's Care Management Institute (CMI) has produced a formal evidence-based Pain Management Guideline, as well as published a Palliative Care Sourcebook which includes guidelines and various clinician tools. Additional materials and resources for symptom control and pain management are available to providers through our online Palliative Care Community. KP is building a strong network of palliative care professionals who communicate, consult, and problem-solve together.

When my own uncle was dying I got to visit him in his home. Because he was home, he could share with me some memorabilia from his life, photo albums, and old newspaper articles he was proud of and he gave me a couple of photos of my own father that I didn't know existed. My own father died suddenly at 59 of a first heart attack, so we did not have that kind of time together in the dying process. That is one of my regrets.

So this week I am celebrating the extension to all Regions of our new Palliative Care Program. The program adds special value at an important time in people's lives.

Let me quote a piece from one of our internal documents about our programs to give you a sense of the working focus of our efforts:

The key features of these palliative care programs include:

Care is person-centered and thereby is culturally competent

Care is comprehensive

Care is holistic and goes beyond the medical domain

Patient/family together is the unit of care

Interdisciplinary team approach addresses the spectrum of needs of patient and family

Focus is on enhancing quality of life

Approach of the team is "values-neutral"; the patient's and family's values are primary, not the team's or any one team member's values.

"Family" is used in a broad sense and includes people who may or may not be related legally or by blood. Often this is elicited by asking: "Who is important to you that you would want us to include in this process?"

Those are great goals and values.So thank you to the pioneers from our care teams and to the caregivers all across Kaiser Permanente who are making palliative care available to our patients. It is exactly the right thing to do.

Well done Palliative Care Teams. Thank you.

Be well.

George

✻ ✻ ✻

Background Note: Freeing Up Nurses to be Nurses

This was also one of my first celebration letters. It celebrates nurses and the work that we have been doing at Kaiser Permanente to help nurses increase the direct time spent with patients. We are doing the work outlined in this letter even more effectively today than when I wrote the letter. It is very much the right thing to do.

Nurses are the heart of every hospital. Nurses anchor most care settings. Patients need the care that only nurses can give.

Too often, in American care settings, nurses end up spending almost all of their time on paperwork and administrative duties, and nurses can't actually get to the patients for enough direct nurse-to-patient care.

We studied that problem, and we have done several things to make that situation better. It was the right thing to do. Our incredible successes in our hospitals on pressure ulcer prevention and quick intervention for hospital infections has been possible in part because our nurses can now spend more time with patients instead of spending their time filling out forms and processing paperwork.

The next letter celebrates both nurses and some of the work we are doing to eliminate administrative distractions so that nurses can provide real care to real patients.

Celebrating Nurses – July 11, 2008

Dear KP Colleagues,

When I had my coronary artery bypass surgery a couple of years ago, one of the things that surprised me was the huge impact that the hospital nurses had on my care and my state of mind.

I have worked in health care for a couple of decades, so I knew and fully appreciated the logistical and operational roles that nurses play in keeping the care system functioning. I had the right intellectual context. What I did not have was the experiential and emotional context.

When you are a patient coming out of major surgery, the world can be an amazingly painful, dysfunctional, unsettling and even sometimes a scary place. You hurt wherever the surgery was done. You are incapacitated. You are wired and tubed and intubated in multiple inconvenient, uncomfortable, unpleasant and awkward ways, and when you are not having the pain killers put you to sleep, you tend to live and concentrate from minute to minute entirely in the minute — focused on your own survival, your own mixture of tubes and medications and measurements and tests. Focused very much on your own concerns about your immediate health status and your future recovery. It is not a good place to be.

What makes the whole process livable are the nurses — the gentle, ever-present, friendly, concerned and caring caregivers who comfort you and inform you and connect you logistically and intellectually with the exact caregiving environment and situation you are in. My nurses encouraged me, reassured me, sympathized and empathized with my pain, sympathized with the IV needles and the catheter and with the fact that coughing hurt my chest so much that I wanted to cry out and somehow get the heck out of the whole situation. But, there is no place to go and nowhere to be but there, and your nurse fills in as your friend and comforter and ally against all the things going wrong in your world.

In the middle of the night — waking to a strange and painful place — the nurses were truly miracles of the moment.

I can clearly remember nurses leaning over the bed and saying, "Hey, you're doing great," — giving me a sense of doing great even when I felt worse than I had ever felt before in my life.

I understood after one day in the recovery unit why patients love nurses and why nurses are the most essential and treasured part of the care world for so many people.

Why do I mention that two year old experience in my weekly letter? I mention it because Kaiser Permanente has been a key part of a wonderful initiative aimed at figuring out how to make nursing even more patient focused and patient centered, and we just released the results of that study to the world.

The project is called Time and Motion — Transforming the Patient Care Environment.

A major goal of the Time and Motion project is to help nurses cut way back on paperwork and spend more time with patients — dispensing medications, running tests, providing care, and giving comfort.

The study collected data from 767 nurses in multiple geographically diverse hospital med-surge units.

The study learned that nurses walk between 2.4 and 3.4 miles per shift. Some nurses walked as far as five miles.

The study learned that paperwork and administration tasks consume more time than direct patient care. Patient care at a face-to-face level consumed about 19.3 percent of nursing shift time — while documentation took over 35 percent of each nurse's time. Medications administration took 17.2 percent of the time.

The nurses and researchers who did the study reached some important conclusions about how nursing should be supported and structured to allow more time with patients, to improve medication accuracy, and to improve patient safety. You can see the study on the News Center.

As a result of the study, Kaiser Permanente and a couple of other leading health care organizations are committed to taking steps to better support nurses in the delivery of care.

This is important work — because it directly addresses key issues and because everyone in health care is learning from the data.

It's even more important work because it helps us support nurses spending time with patients instead of spending time on file folders or paper work. It's a work in progress, but it is a work in progress and that's a good thing.

My own memory of waking in the middle of the night and being with a real person who obviously knew exactly what she or he was doing and who clearly was there to help me with care that I really needed with a level of comfort that I really appreciated tells me that this project is good work to be doing.

So this week I am celebrating the team who did the study and all the nurses at Kaiser Permanente who made the study a success.

Also, I would like to celebrate and again thank the nurses who helped me as my nurses when nursing care was exactly what I needed.

Thank you.

Be well.

George

✿ ✿ ✿

Background Note: Mortality Rates Matter to People Who Die

Mortality rates matter. They matter a lot to the people who die. Some people think of mortality rates as a statistic. Over the years, I have increasingly come to appreciate the fact that mortality rate statistics are actually about real people dying. When I had my own heart surgery, the coronary artery bypass surgery survival rates jumped from being statistics to being my personal odds of not dying. That is, I can tell you, very sobering. And very focusing. At that point, in my own care experience, I was particularly pleased to have helped in a process that put these odds overwhelmingly in my favor. Far too many people talk about mortality rates as though they were a pure statistic or simple competitive metric or even something like a baseball score. Mortality rates are far more than that.

So we measure our mortality rates at Kaiser Permanente, and we do hard work to improve them. We know very clearly and directly that when we do better, people do not die. Real people. Real deaths. It isn't just numbers.

The next letter discusses mortality rates.

Celebrating Our High-Performing Hospital System – August 5, 2011

Dear KP Colleagues,

How do we know that we are doing really good work both as a hospital system and as individual hospitals?

We are one of the largest hospital systems in the country. There are some external indications of how well we are performing. We have won awards for being the most computerized hospitals in America — and maybe the world.

One of our most senior leaders was just elected Chair-Elect of the American Hospital Association — the national organization for all American hospitals. That selection reflects the admiration other hospital leaders across the country hold for the new chair-elect as a person, and as a leader, and it also probably indicates a level of respect from other hospitals for Kaiser Permanente as a high-performing hospital system.

Those are current external indicators. What about internal measures? What information do we look at to get a sense of how well we are doing?

We actually have several levels of internal measures of hospital performance. One of these measures is our patient service and satisfaction scores — the ratings on service given to hospitals by their patients. We survey many thousands of our patients to learn their satisfaction levels with our care.

We will get the official service satisfaction scores for last year in a month or so. I will write about them then.

Those scores influence thinking of a lot of people about how well we do as a system, because those service and satisfaction scores have become the subject of public attention through the news media and various reporting mechanisms.

They also give us an important sense of how our members feel about the care we provide.

Satisfaction levels are important — but they are obviously not the only measure of a hospital. Quality scores are also extremely important for any caregiving organization. So how do we track quality? We measure quality at a number of levels.

One basic ongoing measure of the quality of hospital performance is mortality rates. We measure mortality rates for our patients in each of

126

our regions and each of our hospitals. We track our mortality rate data over time as a tool to help us know how well we are doing in a number of key areas.

We exist to deliver great care. Mortality rates are not a perfect quality measure, but they give us a good tool to see how well we are doing over time as great care sites. We clearly want to know how well we are doing so we can do better. As you can see from these charts, we are continuously improving.

Mortality rate improvements don't just happen.

We know we can improve our mortality rates by continuously making our care better. Infections matter, for example. Infections kill people. We know we can avoid or prevent some infections, respond with blazing speed and great competency to treat other infections, and we can improve our ability to quickly diagnose and respond effectively to other infections.

Every activity component in each of those areas cuts infections, and each improvement drops our mortality rate. Each component of process improvement in our hospitals helps keep more people alive. Improving hospital safety is a wonderful agenda, and it is an extremely important thing to do.

We are learning. We are not perfect. It is a work in progress. We are working hard to be better every day.

So how are we doing?

We don't have the full 2011 dataset yet — but the chart below shows what has been happening to our composite mortality rate by region over the past four years.

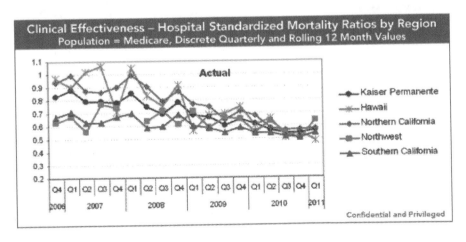

The death rate is dropping. This is a good chart. We are continuously improving our work on hospital safety and best care, and I believe we can expect to see that drop in mortality continue into the future.

As you can see from the chart, last year was better than the year before. People are alive today, and they are at home with their families and their friends today, because we are doing this important work.

Mortality is far from our only measurement of hospital performance. There are many other measurements that we hold dear to our hearts and use in our work of making our hospitals better.

One other interesting measure is worth mentioning in this letter. That other measure gives us one indication of why our mortality rate is going down. It's a composite measure based on the work and the report set done by us for The Joint Commission (TJC). The Joint Commission used to be The Joint Commission on Accreditation of Healthcare Organizations (JCAHO). They simplified the name a couple of years ago. The Joint Commission accredits hospitals all over the country. The accreditation process involves multiple, very solid measures of hospital performance.

The Joint Commission also gets better every year at helping hospitals track performance and improve care. We track care in a number of Joint Commission areas. For the sake of simplicity, their full set of quality measures can be blended into a single chart showing a "composite" quality process score for each hospital.

How are we doing on Joint Commission composite scores? That composite chart is also included in this letter.

Again, I don't have the full set of data for the first half of this year yet — but if you look back over the past four years, the composite Joint Commission scores for quality processes at KP are also moving very much in the right direction.

There are nearly twenty underlying scores that we track for the Joint Commission.

Again — we track each Kaiser Permanente hospital individually on each and every measure. The composite scores are shown below.

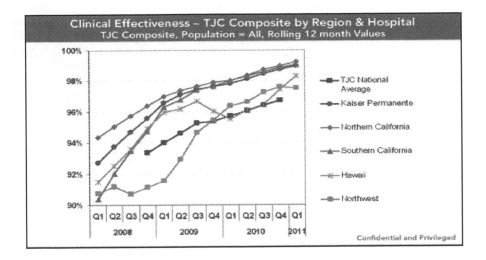

I will update our progress in this entire composite measurement as we go forward into 2012.

For now, for this week, I would like to celebrate everyone in our total hospital care team who is doing the hard work to reduce our mortality rates so successfully — and who is working in all of the categories of performance that combine to give us TJC continuously improving composite report set. We are not perfect, and we are very far from done in our quality journey — but both of these charts show we are moving in a forward direction.

That's a good thing. We exist to take care of people. When our patients need hospital care, these numbers reinforce the fact that we are the right place to be to get that care.

Well done.

Be well.

George

☆ ☆ ☆

Background Note: HIV Patients Benefit Hugely From Team Care – The Environment Benefits When We Are Green

As I said in the last letter, mortality rates matter a lot to people who die.

One area where we have done really good work on significantly reducing mortality rates is in the care given to our HIV-positive patients. We have applied science-based proactive team care to those patients, and we are succeeding at levels that could not be achieved without doing what we are doing.

We have literally dropped our death rate from HIV to half of the national average. We have done that in a process of continuous learning and continuous improvement. We are a lot smarter about how to deliver this care than we were a few years ago, and we continue to get smarter as we continue to provide that care.

We want to share what we learned with the world. We want to share both our success and our learning with the world, so we are now making our HIV programs and our approaches available to anyone in health care who wants to learn them.

The next two letters are about the "HIV Challenge" we issued this year to everyone in America who delivers care. The second letter also includes a challenge to the rest of health care to both reduce pressure ulcers and become more environmentally responsible.

Part of our mission as a caregiving organization is to show the world what is possible. Other people in other care settings can't even aspire to those levels of performance and care quality if they don't know those levels of success are possible. Both of the next two letters celebrate our work in those areas.

Celebrating KP's Global Challenge to Provide Best Care for HIV Patients – January 20, 2012

Dear KP Colleagues,

We plan to challenge the world next week.

Kaiser Permanente caregivers will be in Washington, D.C., challenging the nation to follow our lead in reducing deaths from HIV infections.

We will make the announcement and issue the challenge to the nation next week at the Centers for Medicare and Medicaid Services (CMS) Health Care Innovation Summit.

We have done some amazingly good work on HIV care.

Our combination of team care, best practices, and consistent patient follow-up care has reduced the HIV death rate at Kaiser Permanente to less than half of the national average. We are even 20 percent more effective than the Veterans Administration — another organization that does a great job on HIV care.

We have a higher percentage of patients with treatment adherence — 94 percent median adherence. We also have a higher percent in getting patients care more quickly — at 88 percent. And we have a 38 percent improvement over other sites for earlier diagnosis.

So we are delivering better care.

We won't just be issuing a challenge next week. We will also be offering our help to help other care systems improve their own care.

We will be sharing our tools and our strategies for successful HIV care with the nation. We have learned a lot. We intend to share what we have learned and then encourage all care sites to follow our lead. If that happens, lives will be saved.

One of the things that we are most proud of is the fact that we have not only set a new standard for overall HIV maintenance care — but we also have performed as a care system at a level where there are no differences or disparities in HIV outcomes for patients by race at KP. In the rest of the country, black HIV patients have 15 percent higher mortality rates than whites and are significantly less likely to receive HIV medications. Those disparities do not exist at KP.

Disparities are extremely important to us. We want to deliver disparity-free care. At our annual Kaiser Permanente National Diversity Conference in October of last year, we assembled a specially focused internal summit meeting on disparities. Approximately 100 people attended the Equity Summit.

The summit created a bold set of new goals for Kaiser Permanente on disparities. In a world where care disparities by race, gender, and ethnicity happen far too often, we set a goal of eliminating disparities by ensuring — on a patient-specific basis — that each and all of our patients get the best care.

We track differences in performance by race and ethnicity for 16 NCQA HEDIS categories. Even though our care for all patients is continuously improving, we know that we have areas where differences exist.

Our goal is to make differences disappear.

It's an ambitious goal. But we believe it's an important goal, and it will help us to continuously improve our care.

So my letter this week celebrates our caregivers who will challenge the world next week to produce better care for HIV patients.

My letter also celebrates the KP care leaders at our National Diversity Conference Equity Summit who took the lead to give us a great new set of goals.

Goals make us better. Getting care right for our HIV patients helps remind us who we are.

Be well.

George

✧ ✧ ✧

Celebrating KP Modeling Doing the Right Things for Care Delivery – February 3, 2012

Dear KP Colleagues,

We amazed and impressed and inspired a lot of people in Washington, D.C., last week with our HIV challenge.

When we showed that we had dropped the mortality rate for HIV patients at Kaiser Permanente to half the national average and then challenged the nation to follow in our path, people were suddenly empowered to think differently about what was possible for HIV care.

The response was very warm and highly accepting of our success and our willingness to share what we have learned and our willingness to help other health care organizations and care teams get to similar results.

It was a good week.

We also had a wonderful response from the American Hospital Association about our success in cutting pressure ulcers from almost 3 percent of all patients to under 1 percent over a couple of years.

The AHA wrote a very nice piece that they sent to every AHA-member hospital in the country that talked about what we had done and how we had done it. They also want to feature us in some future meeting settings.

Again, we are serving as a model for the caregivers of America and of the world relative to saving lives and making lives better for our patients.

Pressure ulcers damage and disfigure and kill patients. It is a painful way to die. Cutting those ulcers to very low levels at Kaiser Permanente hospitals is a constant labor of both love and consistent caring. Now other hospitals know it is possible. Possible is a very enabling thing.

Other care sites will not commit and will not even aspire to those ulcer reduction success levels or those HIV mortality reduction rates if they don't think or understand that these levels of successes are actually possible. By showing everyone what is possible, we are changing the way good people think about care in a good way.

We are doing the same thing with environmental sustainability. We aspire to be the world leader in green health care…by being environmentally responsible and adept and effective at multiple levels.

We just released a new set of green purchasing standards, moving the buying of intravenous (IV) medical equipment in what we believe to be the most environmentally responsible way.

We decided to buy IV solution bags that are 100 percent PVC and DEHP free and to buy IV tubing that is also 100 percent free of DEHP. These chemicals have been widely used in medical products and they have been shown to have harmful effects on health and the environment.

We announced that decision to be green in a new way in health care, and the story was picked up by close to 100 media outlets, including The Washington Post and the San Francisco Chronicle.

Again, by changing what we buy, we gave people in health care a new way to think about what could and can and should be done in another important area of care.

Green is good.

We only have this one planet. We need to take care of this planet individually and collectively. Making environmentally safer purchases is a step in that direction.

I suspect others will follow our lead there, as well, now that we have gone down that path.

So that's my celebration for this week. We continue to do important things that help the rest of the world redefine what is possible and create their own paths to saving lives and saving the environment.

We have a wonderful opportunity to make a difference for our patients by doing things well and also to make a difference to the world by sharing and teaching the important things that we do really well. That's a good thing to do. It is definitely worth doing.

So thank you to our HIV team leaders and thank you to all of our caregivers who work with every patient in our hospitals every day to keep those pressure ulcers from ruining lives and thank you to our green team for coming up with another way for us to help protect the planet.

Well done.

Be well.

George

＊ ＊ ＊

Background Note: Saving Lives with Cancer Care

We save a lot of lives with our cancer care programs at Kaiser Permanente. We don't just look at cancer as a reactive medical crisis. We look at cancer as an entire care agenda — beginning with prevention, anchored on early detection, and then crowned with great care when patients are in need of great care.

Our genius thinking on cancer care relates to early detection. We set a macro goal for Kaiser Permanente of having the lowest number and lowest percentage of cancers get to stages 3 and 4.

Late stage cancers are very hard to cure. Early stage cancers have much higher cure rates. So we work very hard with our detection programs to detect cancers early. We have the highest quality scores in the country on several categories of early detection.

We also work very hard to cure the cancers we do detect. Unlike many solo practice doctors who can have a very hard time keeping up with best practices and delivering consistent optimal care, we have our own internal collection of brilliant oncologists who make sure that we keep up on cancer care treatment effectiveness and best practices. We have hundreds of cancer protocols that have significantly improved cancer care.

We also do a lot of cancer research. With nearly 60,000 total cancer patients, we have over 6,000 patients in nearly 100 clinical trials. We published 178 articles last year on our cancer research. Most people have no clue that we have one of the largest and best cancer research agendas in health care.

The next letter talks about our total cancer agenda. The letter points out that we win on the detection scales and we also do really well on the survivability scales for patients with cancer.

Compared to national averages for cancer care results, we do better on our survival rates for several cancers. Even our lung cancer survival rates, for example, are significantly better than the national average. Our melanoma survival rates are among the best in the world, and our breast cancer survival rates at 95 percent are significantly better than the national average reported by SEER (Surveillance, Epidemiology, and End Results) at 89 percent.

This next letter celebrates that entire package of care. It's good to be good at cancer care. Cancer care is hugely important to people with cancer.

Celebrating Our Cancer Care Successes – July 6, 2012

Dear KP Colleagues,

Cancer care saves a lot of lives at Kaiser Permanente.

Everyone knows that Kaiser Permanente does a great job of taking care of people with chronic conditions. We are not perfect — and we are on a path of continuous improvement in many areas — but we do a very good job of helping people with key chronic conditions improve their health and minimize the levels of damage done by those diseases.

We actually lead the nation on quite a few HEDIS quality scores relative to chronic condition care. We do a great job of managing blood cholesterol levels for diabetics. We are number one in hypertension control. We are number one in osteoporosis screening.

We very much want our patients who have chronic conditions to have the most minimal suffering and damage from their diseases, and we use systems-supported team care to achieve those goals. We tend to be successful.

We have even reduced the mortality rate for our HIV patients to half of the national average.

We also are a leader in hospital safety. We have some of the lowest levels of both sepsis deaths and deeply damaging pressure ulcers in the world. People who are hospitalized in other hospitals are, on average, twice as likely to be damaged or die from those conditions.

We have won multiple awards and recognitions for our hospital care. So Kaiser Permanente care delivery successes in those areas are not invisible. We do, however, have another whole category of care where our successes have not been very visible to the world. People outside our walls do not have a good sense at all of how well we do on cancer care.

So how well do we do?

We have some very solid results there, as well. We are saving a lot of lives with our cancer care.

We are a world leader for early detection. That is very intentional.

One of our underlying goals as an organization for a number of years has been to lead care delivery in having the lowest percent of cancers getting to stages 3 and 4.

Why did we set that early detection goal? For obvious medical reasons.

Stage 1 cancers are usually treatable. We can generally save lives relatively easily with stage 1 cancers. Stage 2 cancers are still treatable, but more patients die when cancers get to stage 2.

Stages 3 and 4 cancers are the most dangerous. The risks are clearly higher for those patients.

So that's why we set a deliberate goal for ourselves of having the very fewest cancers getting to stages 3 and 4.

How do we achieve that goal? In very practical ways. We are focused heavily on early detection. We send out millions of colon cancer detection kits to our members a year. I am at an age at which I get these kits regularly, along with regular follow-up reminders and even an occasional direct email from my doctor reminding me when I haven't done what I should be doing for the cause of prevention.

How well is that program working? You can go to this video link to hear one of our patients talking about how well that approach worked for him.

We actually lead the country on that particular early detection process, and we can see a declining death rate from colon cancer as a result.

In fact, we just did a study with our Southern California Region that showed the numbers of colon cancers we are detecting at stage 0 or 1 has risen by 28 percent to 41 percent. That same study showed that our number of late-stage colon cancer detections has come down by 32 percent to only 13 percent.

Thirteen percent is still a very serious number — particularly if you are one of the 13 percent. But the truth is that we had 32 percent of our colon cancer patients get to late-stage before we started our aggressive early detection program.

That early detection work has been helped significantly by our "Proactive Office Encounter" system. I have celebrated that system in earlier letters. The Proactive Office Encounter has tools that give our care teams triggers, prompts, and reminders that make every single patient visit for any purpose a potential prevention visit. Southern California also pioneered that lovely systematic "proactive" work, and it is saving lives.

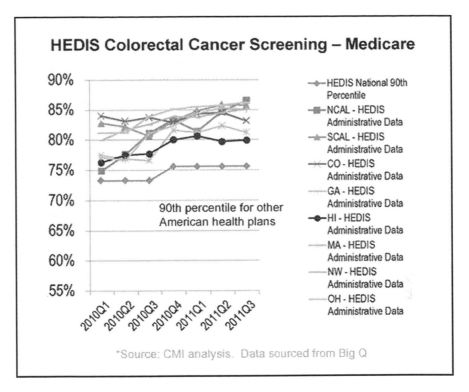

The lowest colorectal cancer screening line shown on the above chart isn't us. It is the 90th percentile for all other health plans in America. All of our regions exceed that 90th percentile for screenings.

We also lead the country in breast cancer screening. We could well do more mammograms than any care organization in the world. We also use reminders to help trigger mammograms for patients who come to our care sites to get care for other conditions. We even have a mammography van that goes out to the patients. We pioneered that idea in Hawaii.

We have top HEDIS scores in the country and in each region for mammography.

We also have excellent cervical cancer screening rates. Our Pap test numbers are very high. We are also detecting those cancers at an earlier stage because we emphasize getting the tests.

Early detection for each of those cancers also help patient survival.

Stage 1 cervical cancer is obviously much more curable than 3 or stage 4 cervical cancer.

We also are very focused on helping patients quit smoking. Our overall KP smoking rates are now close to half the national average.

Not smoking helps keep lung cancers from starting and then getting to stages 3 and 4. Curing lung cancer is incredibly difficult. Preventing lung cancer can happen if people stop smoking — so we strongly support people giving up smoking.

We are also encouraging walking as an activity for all patients. How is walking related to cancer? There are studies that show that colon cancer, breast cancer, and prostate cancer risks are all 25 percent or more lower for people who walk more than 30 minutes a day, five days a week. We are not alone. The American Cancer Society also encourages physical activity for cancer protection.

We encourage walking for multiple reasons — and both cancer prevention and cancer recovery are included in those reasons.

Overall, our early detection agendas are solid and effective. We believe that we are saving a lot of lives for cancer patients who would be gone today if their cancer had not been detected until a later stage.

So those are the early detection and prevention agendas. How are we doing on actual treatment for the cancers our patients have once they are detected?

Again — the numbers look very good.

We just did another study that looked at our Southern California database. We compared our outcomes to the care outcomes for those same cancers released by SEER. SEER stands for Surveillance, Epidemiology, and End Results, and it is the official national cancer measurement system.

What did we learn?

For breast cancer, across all patients with that cancer, the SEER study showed that 89 percent of the cancer patients in the country survived five years.

How did we do?

Our study showed us that at Kaiser Permanente, 95 percent of the women with breast cancer were still alive after five years.

We did better.

What about colon cancer? For the country, SEER data showed that 65 percent of colon cancer patients are still alive in five years.

What about Kaiser Permanente?

Again — we did better.

Our data from the Southern California study shows that 75 percent of our colon cancer patients in the region are still alive after five years. Our goal is to move that number up even higher.

For melanoma patients, the SEER survival rate for the country is 91 percent. Our Southern California study showed that the survival rate for Kaiser Permanente melanoma patients was 99 percent.

Team care, early detection, quick response, and best medical science all combine to bring that success level to a very good place.

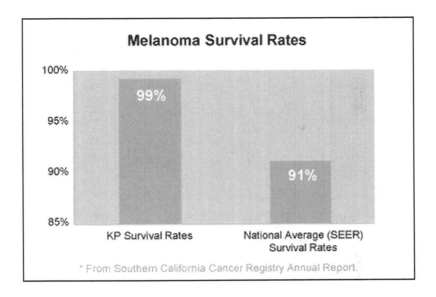

What about lung cancer?

Lung cancer is really hard. Lung cancer is a very difficult cancer to treat. Lung cancer is usually fatal. That is one of the reasons we try so hard to help smokers quit smoking. We really need better lung cancer prevention because — for all health care systems — the cure is so very hard to realize.

For lung cancer, the national SEER survival rate for cancer patients is slightly under 16 percent. How did we do? Better.

Our current success rate from the Southern California study is now 19 percent.

Nineteen percent is a tough number. We are working hard to figure out how to make it better. The national five-year lung cancer survival average for all care sites in this country who report data to SEER is 15.9

percent. That is an even tougher number. We clearly need to get everyone who smokes to stop smoking so we can reduce deaths from that cancer.

What does all of that data say about our overall cancer care? We have some very impressive numbers. We are doing some things very well. We need to build on our strengths. We are learning, and we are continuously improving. We are number one in the country for many aspects of chronic care. We are number one for many aspects of care connectivity. We are among the very best care teams in the world at multiple levels of prevention and intervention.

We also are aiming at being the very best in cancer care. Many of our cancer care outcomes clearly equal or exceed the national SEER average. We want to do even better. We have great technology, great care teams, and we can keep up with evolving and improving medical science in a systematic way that is almost impossible to do for solo practice physicians.

We also participate in a number of clinical trials. We are moving the science for cancer care forward through those trials. We currently have more than 64,000 total patients in clinical trials for various medical conditions. About a dozen of our clinical trials involve cancer patients. Roughly, 6,000 Kaiser Permanente patients are in cancer clinical trials.

I will write about some of our cancer research and our cancer care best practices in another weekly letter. I started to write about those points for this letter, but this letter is getting to be a very long letter, so I will save those topics for later.

So that is our macro cancer care strategy. We start with detection. We are focused very heavily on our goal of keeping cancers for our patients from getting to stages 3 and 4. That is a good thing to do.

And we want to be sure that if cancer gets to the late stages, we are the right place to be for people who have that problem in their lives.

The melanoma numbers are very encouraging.

Ninety-nine percent survival is a very good score when we are talking about mortality levels.

So my letter this week celebrates our entire cancer care team — the people who prevent, detect, intercept, research, and treat cancer at Kaiser Permanente. We are, like all cancer care settings, far from perfect — but we are doing really good work and we are continuously improving.

That's exactly what our members deserve when they trust us with their care.

Let me make one final point.

When we look at cancer care, we need to look at mortality rates.

Mortality rates are more than just numbers. People are involved. Real people. Mortality rates matter a lot to the people who die.

So let's keep bringing the mortality rates down.

Well done.

Be well.

George.

✵ ✵ ✵

Background Note: We Are a Care Team — So Team Care Needs To Be Something We Do Really Well

Team care is extremely important to us at Kaiser Permanente. We are, at our core, a care team. We know that team care can make care better for large numbers of our patients. We know that when patients have multiple health conditions, team care can be golden. We know that when patients have complex care needs, their care takes a patient-focused care response, and one of our goals is to make that actual complexity invisible to the patient. We want a high level of care coordination to be part of the core skillset of our care team.

The rest of the country is looking at creating Accountable Care Organizations (ACO's) and patient-focused Medical Homes. In some respects, we are the care approach that those new care design models are trying to emulate.

We are committed as an organization to work in teams to provide team-based patient care. We used a team approach to build our electronic medical record. We use team approaches every day on the front lines of our organization. We have more than 90,000 of our employees now working in unit-based teams, each team focusing on improving our care safety and our care delivery at the frontline site of care. We believe that no one in the world has more of their frontline health care workers in unit-based teams.

Team care is us.

One of my celebration letters featured a patient who had experienced our team care and wrote a letter to me describing her experiences.

Celebrating Team Care - October 8, 2010

Dear KP Colleagues,

I just read a letter from one of our patients who has cancer.

She is recovering. She feels very good about her care.

The thing that struck me most about her letter was that she said that she has received care from a team — and that felt good.

She said that over the course of her diagnosis, consultations, tests, scans, therapies, surgeries, and multiple treatments, she has been counting the number of Kaiser Permanente caregivers who took care of her — and she stopped counting at 296.

That is a lot of people. Doctors, nurses, therapists, technicians, phlebotomists, pharmacists, medication managers — she was helped by a lot of folks at Kaiser Permanente — and what she really appreciated was the fact that the whole group of KP caregivers functioned as a team and everyone had her information and everyone knew what her immediate care needs were. She appreciated how each caregiver fit together with every other caregiver to create a total team — and she felt the team was focused on her.

We take our teamness for granted at Kaiser Permanente. We know that we have aligned caregivers, a single medical record, shared diagnosis, shared tests and medical information, and a philosophy of caring for our patients in patient-focused teams.

We should not take that teamness for granted. It is a very special thing.

The daughter of a very dear friend of mine is currently going through a bout of medical care in a non-KP city. She also has a slightly complex care issue, and diagnosis is proving difficult.

She has now been seen by seven different medical practices.

The medical practices who are seeing her are coordinating absolutely nothing.

They are not sharing information.

They are not sharing test results.

They are not communicating with one another in any way.

They function in isolated silos.

Each time she goes to a new practice, they start the tests all over. They don't share lab data, and they don't even share tentative diagnoses.

She just had to give an attorney power of attorney to go to each medical practice who has seen her to get a full set of the paper records that each clinic has in their files about her and her condition.

When she gets them all together, she intends to give them all to an eighth care site to see if they can figure out a diagnosis that can help her resolve some issues of intense pain and impaired functionality that she has.

The point of my letter isn't that she has a hard to diagnose medical problem. Unfortunately, that happens.

The point is that she has been completely truncated in her attempts to get any of her caregivers to communicate in any way with any other caregiver.

They all have paper medical records. The medical records do not interact with each other. They don't blend together automatically to create a single full picture of her condition.

There is no care team in her town — and she needs team care.

So when I hear her frustration and I hear my friend share intense unhappiness about her daughter's uncoordinated, unlinked, and unconnected care — and then I get a letter from one of our Kaiser Permanente patients about her fully linked and fully connected care who stopped counting her care team at 296 caregivers — I have a very clear reminder of why we are so special.

So my celebration this week is the 296 caregivers who linked up so well that our patient felt like she was the focus of a team of people who were really focused on her.

It's good to do team care well.

Be well.

George

* * *

Background Note: We Hold Major Internal Conferences Regularly to Learn from Ourselves

One of the very best ways of learning at Kaiser Permanente is to get people who are kindred spirits together and to hold a conference with great topics, great speakers, and great interaction between conference participants.

When a conference is really well done, as much learning happens in the hallway interaction between the participants as it does in the lectures, speeches, seminars and the panel discussions onstage.

As a collectively learning organization, we love our conferences. We learn a lot at our conferences that we couldn't possibly learn if everyone just stayed in their care sites every day of the year.

We hold four major national conferences and two more focused topic-centered conferences every year. One of the major conferences deals with quality. One deals with diversity. Another conference deals with community benefit.

We also hold a major conference — The Permanente Executive Leadership Summit — for all of our medical leaders to optimize all of the evolving opportunities that exist in health care at Kaiser Permanente.

In addition to those major conferences, we hold a smaller innovation conference to celebrate our progress in innovation, and we convene a smaller compliance conference to teach our people how to comply with the contact stream of new laws and regulations. We literally have had 14,000 pages of new regulations and rules written in just the last two years that apply to Kaiser Permanente — so the people at the compliance conference have some heavy lifting to do.

I tend to write celebration letters about each of the four major conferences. The next letter celebrated a recent quality conference.

Celebrating Continuous Quality Learning – Real and Virtual – July 29, 2011

Dear KP Colleagues,

The head of the Institute for Healthcare Improvement taught a seminar last week on "Ten New Rules to Redesign and Improve Care."

Where did she teach that class?

Kaiser Permanente.

Three experts taught a session last week on "One Size Does Not Fit All — Using Population Tailoring to Address Disparities."

Where did that session happen?

Kaiser Permanente.

Two other experts taught a session on "The Use of Virtual Visits to Improve the Management of Patients in Orthopedics and Other Specialties."

Where did that session happen?

Kaiser Permanente.

We just held another amazing annual National Quality Conference. The agenda is located at the conference website.

The conference had sessions like "How to Eliminate Disparities in Diabetes Care and Hypertension Management in Chinese KP Members."

And "Changing the Culture of Infant Feeding."

And "Using Exercise as a Vital Sign."

And "Targeting Zero Health Care Associated Infections in the NICU."

Experts spoke at session after session for two full days. We had 38 breakout sessions and another 21 supplemental sessions — all with great topics.

The conference was attended by five hundred Kaiser Permanente caregivers in person. Another twenty-five hundred caregivers attended electronically at 75 remote Kaiser Permanente locations.

The conference was recorded — and the sessions will now be available to all of our care teams virtually.

If you get a chance, take the time to look at that website, and read the list of topics. These are the kinds of topics that we would want as a learning agenda for the caregivers who take care of our own families and the people we love.

Our own KP goal is to be the best quality care organization in the world. Quality doesn't just happen.

Quality isn't something that just gets handed to anyone. Quality is a quest and a journey, and the path to quality involves a commitment to continuous learning.

Continuous learning is the best learning. Getting better and smarter every day is the best approach to learning.

We know that we are delivering really solid — in many cases best — care at Kaiser Permanente today. We also know that the science of care improves and changes all the time and that we get smarter every day about improving the process of care.

So we are building getting smarter into our care support toolkit.

Our electronic medical library is one of our steps in the continuous learning process. That library is unique to us. Every KP caregiver can get real-time access to the full set of medical research journals, best practices, and recommended care publications. Our electronic care library is a care support tool — built by our care team — that doesn't really exist any-where else on the planet.

Our goal is to learn and teach and to deliver great care. The National Quality Conference is a place where we both learn and teach.

The really solid team of quality people who put this conference together — and the absolutely stellar set of presenters — have again moved us down the path to continuous improvement in a really solid way.

So this week I am celebrating our National Quality Conference — and I am celebrating the fact that all of the people of Kaiser Permanente — the entire care team — can now get access to this solid and timely set of learning opportunities.

Really good stuff.

Well done.

Be well.

George

✲ ✲ ✲

Background Note: Learning Can Be Learned As a Community

We strongly believe in collaborative learning.

We exist to benefit our members, our patients, and our communities. We don't pay a cash dividend as an organization. We pay a "mission dividend." We also exist to provide great value to the employers and governmental agencies that use us to provide health coverage and health care to their beneficiaries and their employees. We don't have shareholders. We do have very important stakeholders, and we will not succeed without providing great value to all of those stakeholders.

Part of our mission is to make the communities we are in better, healthier, and better informed about key topics relating to care and health. The next letter deals with a couple of our conferences on those topics — including our community benefit conferences.

Again — one of our strengths as an organization is the collaborative learning opportunities that are created by our wide range, scope, and scale of care sites and activities. We are actually bigger as a total care system than 42 states and 135 countries. We figure out a lot of really good things to do in various sites across that macro care system, and one of our strengths is that we can learn things and then share what we learn. Getting people together in a conference of shared best practices can help us benefit from the huge learning asset that inherently exists because we have so many teams of people in so many places.

This letter celebrates several of those conferences and some of our shared learning times. The touch-screen tool kit and technology that was mentioned in this letter was being tested a couple of years ago by Kaiser Permanente in care sites before it was released to the general public. You may recognize the piece of equipment we were testing in a prerelease setting by the functionality it contains.

Celebrating Our Collaborative Learning Times -
November 12, 2010

Dear KP Colleagues,

Three weeks ago, we brought about 300 members of our community benefit and community service team to San Francisco to share best practices and to celebrate the successes of our Community Benefit programs.

It was a great meeting.

We shared a lot of information.

Two weeks ago, we brought about 550 of our diversity and cultural competency team members from around the country to a meeting in Los Angeles — Hollywood, to be specific — to share learnings and best practices relative to delivering optimal care in the most intelligent and appropriate ways to our wonderfully diverse membership and patient population.

That also was a great meeting. Super speakers. Solid sessions. High energy interactions between committed and focused people.

One week ago, we brought together about 200 of our IT leaders from across the country — physicians, IT managers and analysts, and process improvement experts, who talked about the things we are doing to make the largest non-governmental electronic medical record and support system in the world a great tool to support care.

Again, it was a great conference. High energy, very creative, with solid speakers, and a time of real learning.

Each of those meetings had a set of off-site video links set up and each also set up its own small on-site exhibit hall. Great exhibits. At the IT meeting, I saw a new hand-held touch-screen device that had a lunch-pail-like handle on top, a great and clear touch-screen on the front, a bar code scanner on one end, and a video camera on the other end — so our caregiver could see the patient record on the screen, then use the device to scan medications, verify patient ID, and actually send an image of the patient (like a suture or a bruise) by video for a consult with an off-site caregiver.

It's an amazing piece of equipment — currently being tested as part of our strategy of continuously improving our connectivity and technology.

This week — continuing to build momentum — we held our annual Permanente Executive Leadership Summit (PELS) in Washington, D.C.

It was a great conference.

We not only had more than 150 of our own physician leaders at the conference sharing information about top quality care and best practices, we also had senior medical leaders from several of the other top medical groups in the country.

Mayo, Geisinger, HealthPartners, and Intermountain Health Care all sent both observers and speakers to the conference.

Nancy-Ann DeParle, the White House Director for Health Care Reform, opened the Monday morning PELS session with a talk about care quality, care safety, and the leadership role Kaiser Permanente is playing in helping the country understand what right care should look like.

Nancy-Ann also told the folks at PELS that President Obama had deeply appreciated the great care our Kaiser Permanente care team in Hawaii had given his own grandmother, and she said he had recognized us for that care.

What is very special about that care is that we were providing great care to his grandmother long before she was the grandmother of a president of the United States. She received great care because she was our KP member and patient — not because she had a famous relative.

PELS was a huge success. PELS is extremely important to KP because we are a learning organization — and we need PELS to share what we have learned.

If we learn something in one site and it is done in just that site, that is good but that is not great.

Great is when we learn things and share what we learn.

PELS did exactly that.

You can find more information on each of our recent meetings here:

Community Benefit Summit

National Diversity Conference

IT Summit (on IdeaBook)

Permanente Executive Leadership Summit.

It has been a good month for KP get-togethers.

My letter this week celebrates the KP leaders and teams who have worked so hard to make our shared learning times so successful.

Thank you.

Well done.

Be well.

George

✻ ✻ ✻

Background Note: Patient-Focused Care Teams Can Do Great Things – Including Safely Delivering The World's Only Living Octuplets

We believe in team care.

Sometimes only a team can get the care job done. The next letter thanked the care team at one of our hospitals for delivering the world's only surviving set of octuplets. Delivering eight babies from one mother was a huge clinical and functional challenge. We did not provide the fertility treatments used by the mother. That fact was disclosed by the mother and became a matter of public knowledge, so I am not violating the HIPAA Privacy Rule in any way by mentioning it here. So we were not part of the fertility process. We were, however, a huge part of the survival process. We did actually deliver the eight babies. The truth is that it took many hours of preparation and planning and rehearsal to accomplish what no care team anywhere in the world has ever done before — deliver octuplets who all survived. Team care worked. Our care team did great work.

The next letter thanked that care team and celebrates their success.

Celebrating Extraordinary Care Under Extraordinary Circumstances – February 6, 2009

Dear KP Colleagues,

Our medical professionals at Bellflower Medical Center in Los Angeles did an amazing thing on January 26th. They delivered eight babies in five minutes from one mother.

They did a flawless job.

Our team knew that the lives of seven tiny babies were at stake. So the team practiced, drilled, rehearsed, prepared, choreographed, and then performed brilliantly.

Everyone at Kaiser Permanente should be proud of the excellent care our team delivered.

The whole process started several months ago when we learned that one of our members was near the end of her first trimester and expecting multiple babies.

Our physician leaders at Bellflower pulled together 52 professionals: three obstetricians, two anesthesiologists, seven neonatologists, seven respiratory therapists, 11 NICU RNs, 13 labor and delivery RNs and nine other medical health professionals to make sure we were prepared to bring these babies into the world. We also set aside four delivery rooms, each with two infant warmers and two infant transporters — the most any one room can accommodate.

The team drilled and practiced the delivery for weeks. They even used one of the mechanical training mannequins that I wrote about in a weekly letter last year to improve the team's coordination. The training dummy can ordinarily deliver either one baby or twins, so eight babies was an entirely new use of that particular tool.

Some staff members were assigned one of the first seven letters of the alphabet (A-G), so that each baby would have its own care coordinator in those first critical minutes of life.

Seven letters seemed like enough based on the ultrasounds. But as we all now know, Baby H decided to arrive unannounced. The Bellflower delivery team relied on one another and their training, to make room for one more in the midst of this nearly unprecedented event.

All eight babies are now breathing on their own and are the longest surviving octuplets in American history.

Our media team tells me that there have been nearly 8,500 stories on the octuplets since their birth last week. While this media coverage has not been without controversy, our role is to provide the best care and counsel to all of our patients while respecting their right to privacy — and that's what we did in this situation. Amid the world-wide attention that this story received, our team has stayed focused on delivering the best care possible.

We have stayed true to our mission.

The births at Bellflower reinforce the importance of training and teamwork — so that we are always prepared for any patient that comes through our doors.

So this week I am celebrating the excellent team of caregivers at Bellflower who helped deliver a world record-tying eight babies and who are doing great work to protect and care for each of those tiny little babies and their mother.

I am also celebrating the similar teams across Kaiser Permanente who are taking care of hundreds of premature infants and their families with the same professional dedication.

My own grandson born last year weighed two pounds and nine ounces. He is now doing very well. I know how much skill it takes to deliver care to one tiny baby.

Our Bellflower team is now taking care of eight tiny infants and showing the world what a great medical team can do.

Thank you Bellflower.

Be well.

George

* * *

Background Note – Teamness Is A State of Mind As Well As A Process

My weekly letters often celebrate various Kaiser Permanente care teams. The next very early letter talks about a team of KP folks who are not delivering care as a team but they are, instead, literally paddling a boat as a team.

We sponsor dragon boat competitions. We believe that physical activity is a fundamental behavior needed for good health — and we support and endorse activity at a very clear level through our support of these races and some of the teams in these races.

We are, in fact, the chief sponsor of the San Francisco event. The international Dragon Boat Races in San Francisco Bay are sponsored entirely by us. We also have several dragon boat teams of our own.

I personally love the dragon boat races. I have written a couple of weekly letters about the races and about our teams. This letter is actually a broader celebration of teamness and talks about those races as an example of why it is so good to be a team.

Celebrating Teams – December 26, 2008

Dear KP Colleagues,

As the year draws to a close, I have been thinking back to some of our achievements and accomplishments this year. We have made a lot of progress in multiple areas. Our research has made care better for people across the planet. Our new systems are giving us new tools to use to improve care and service.

Our public policy work is helping people in Washington and state capitals rethink how care can be delivered and should be delivered.

We have a lot of things working together very nicely to move us in good directions.

Our whole agenda reminds me a little of an experience I had a few months ago with the members of our dragon boat team at the Kaiser Permanente International Dragon Boat Races held in San Francisco Bay.

We sponsor the tournament, and we have several teams competing. Our team members work incredibly hard — and want very much to win — but they tell me that winning is only one part of the joy of being a dragon boat team member. The real point, the paddlers tell me, is winning as a team. And "having a great race" as a team.

This year, I asked several team members exactly what it meant to "have a great race."

What they told me was that having a great race is about teamness — functioning as a team — paddling as a team — the joy of being in sync as a team. Complete sync.

Twenty people paddle those long skinny boats. Ten on a side. The drummer on the bow beats a beat and the paddlers paddle in perfect synchronization — up, down, back, up, down, back, etc., for the full length of the race. Dragon boat racing is completely and entirely a team sport. The team functions as a unit. When the boat is truly in the groove, the paddles move in perfect harmony with each other. It's lovely to see — and team members tell me it feels very good and very right to do.

I had one team member about my age tell me, "Sometimes for the last fifty yards, I am so tired I can hardly lift the paddle — but I know that the team needs me to be there in perfect stroke with everyone else on the team. So I keep on the stroke even when my arms are so heavy it's hard to lift the paddle."

Another team member told me, "When we do it right — when we are all in perfect sync and we feel the boat moving through the water as we make each stroke, it feels like we are running the perfect race."

Another team member told me — "I do it for the sheer joy of that sense of being a part of the team. It's about being a team. We often win — and that's good — but the real lift to me comes from running the perfect team race, not just winning. It's a team reward and a team effort."

I found that to be an interesting insight. Being part of a team that does everything well and in sync can be an end in itself.

Reminiscing a bit at the end of the year, I have a feeling that that is sort of what we want to do with our own larger team and with our local teams at Kaiser Permanente. We — more than anyone in health care — have the opportunity to be the perfect system. We have all the pieces — doctors, nurses, lab technicians, radiology technicians, pharmacists, schedulers, phone advisors, health educators, health aides, counselors, therapists, and every other category of caregiver. Our team has sales, marketing, finance, human resources, information technology, legal, and other categories of professionals who help us to operate a strong business that serves our customers, members, and communities. We are all one team. We are putting together both local care teams and a sort of health care mega boat — using systems that give only us "all of the information, about all of the patients, all of the time" — to deliver care, improve care and promote health in ways that splintered, siloed, unorganized and perversely incented non Kaiser Permanente health care organizations can't begin to do.

I keep saying that Kaiser Permanente is a great place to be, and this is a great time to be here. We have a chance to be the very best — the best for patients and our communities and the best for everyone on the team — if we collectively take this opportunity to work as a team to run — or paddle — the perfect race.

My sense at the races every year is that our dragon boat teams understand that possibility and the dragon boat team members know how good it can feel to really get it right.

So I am celebrating both those teams and the whole idea of us all getting it right. Winning is wonderful. Winning by collectively doing the perfect race is even better.

Have a great week. We had a great year.

Be well.

George

✿ ✿ ✿

Background Note: The Wildfires Gave Us Another Unexpected Chance To Use Our New Electronic Care Support Tools

One of the dragon boat teams in the San Francisco races is made up of 20 blind paddlers. Their boat is called "Blind Ambition." Another boat is made up of cancer survivors. They race as "Team Inspire." They do inspire. In each case, in each boat, they function as a team.

We also saw some very inspirational team work when the wildfires raged through Southern California a couple of years ago and forced us to deliver care in innovative ways using our electronic toolkits to help members whose lives were disrupted by the fire.

We have sent caregiver teams to various disaster zones around the country and around the world a number of times. We still have caregivers periodically supporting the care needs of the people from the New Orleans flood. We have helped in a number of settings. I have written weekly letters celebrating some of those efforts where we have been helping people in remote care sites. In this case, however, the disaster came to us. We needed to be our own disaster response team.

The letter is longer than my usual letters — but it tells the story of how the new database care support tools and our electronic medical record continuous availability can help us meet patient needs as a team even when natural disasters strike.

Celebrating KP's Heroes – October 26, 2007

Dear KP Colleagues,

This week I would like to thank and celebrate our care teams and staff affected by the tragic wildfires raging through Southern California. This is not the letter I planned to write this week, but this is a very good time to acknowledge and thank the Kaiser Permanente teams who are caring for our members and community through this horrible disaster. Many employees and physicians are taking care of patients despite their own personal adversity. Their commitment and pure caregiving spirit has been in a number of cases literally heroic.

Many of our people live in the areas devastated by the fires. Many have suffered personal losses. Quite a few employees have been forced to leave their own homes. In too many cases, our people have actually lost their homes to the fires. Yet, Kaiser Permanente facilities out of the fires' paths remain open and we continue to provide care for members and patients from the areas affected by the fire. How could that happen? It is happening because Kaiser Permanente teams quickly mobilized to back-fill positions for those unable to make it into work. We have been very successful in doing that. The spirit of our caregivers is evident.

Our efforts to help have extended beyond direct care delivery. As schools and day care facilities throughout San Diego County began to close, Kaiser Permanente teams quickly established emergency child care centers at four KP facilities. Throughout this week, those centers will provide employees and physicians with 24-hour emergency child care so they can come in to work and continue to care for members and patients. One youngster was overheard asking, "Is this a school? I like this better than my school. I want to stay here."

Other displaced employees are staying at hotels near our facilities so they can be sure to make it into work and continue to deliver care and service to our patients. An interregional KP meeting planned for San Diego was cancelled due to the fires, so our staff arranged to use the hotel rooms we had already reserved to house new moms who were ready for discharge from the hospital, but who lived in evacuated areas, and could not return to their homes.

Kaiser Permanente is also making emergency financial assistance available to KP employees and physicians affected by the wildfires.

This is a very good time to have electronic medical records. Many areas in Southern California have been evacuated and some of our facilities in San Diego County have had to close temporarily. In cases where the fires have forced us to close facilities, our physicians and nurses are using KP HealthConnect® to reach out to patients whose appointments have been cancelled to make sure their needs are met. They are communicating with members by telephone and secure e-mail. Because nearly all Southern California members have KP HealthConnect electronic health records, we are able to direct them to other open Kaiser Permanente facilities with the knowledge that when they arrived for care, their medical record will be electronically available to our caregivers as needed. In the case of fire, paper medical records are often lost forever. Our electronic, medical records are safe and available.

Members who are unable to access their regular Kaiser Permanente pharmacy are also still able to have prescriptions filled at any pharmacy (including non-Kaiser Permanente pharmacies) by presenting their ID and member record number.

Some of our bilingual physicians in Southern California have gone on Spanish-language television to inform the community about the health hazards of smoke for children, the elderly, and those with asthma, heart disease or chronic health conditions.

The Southern California Region has worked with the San Diego community and other provider organizations in the areas impacted to provide care to those needing medical services. So for those people who need care, but who do not have insurance coverage, teams have implemented a system to provide our Medical Financial Assistance Program in the areas affected by the fires — ensuring that those who need care receive it.

As part of our standard disaster planning agenda, we have stockpiled some "disaster relevant" equipment. We used one item of that equipment in response to the fires — a large hospital tent. We prepared our care site for potential patient overcrowding at the San Diego Medical Center main campus by setting up a 40-foot dome tent in the parking lot to triage patients. When evacuations kept staff from returning to their homes, the tent and available cots were also used to provide some exhausted staff members a place to sleep. The good news was, we did not need to use the tent for patients…but it was ready and in place if needed.

In addition, Kaiser Permanente has pledged $250,000 for immediate and long-term needs associated with the Southern California wildfires. We have given $100,000 to the American Red Cross Disaster Relief Fund to provide shelter, food, counseling, and other assistance to victims of the fires. An additional $150,000 is earmarked for long-term fire recovery relief as needs emerge.

I could write a much longer letter on this point. With a disaster of this scope and scale, there are many heroes — from individual firefighters battling the fires to federal agencies providing disaster relief to people affected by the fires. We are grateful to all of them for their work. For now, I want to specifically applaud the many Kaiser Permanente heroes — from our caregivers to our call center representatives and from our receptionists to our radiology techs — in Southern California. Our people are all at work helping our members, the community, and each other through this tragedy with compassionate care and understanding.

Be well,

George

✳ ✳ ✳

Background Note: Is it Better to Practice on Real Patients or to Practice on Robots?

Teams in the world of athletics don't usually just show up on the field for the very first time as a team on game day and somehow play the game. Most teams practice as a team in a practice setting before the actual event. Athletic teams all know the value and the benefit of practicing.

Health care teams, by contrast, haven't traditionally done a lot of practicing. Many care teams in many settings never practice at all. They don't even run drills in many care settings. We are learning to use a different approach at Kaiser Permanente. The weekly letter about us delivering the octuplets made the point that we actually did several dress rehearsals as a team as practice for those births. Those were not our first dress rehearsals. We also increasingly do dress rehearsals for "code blues" in our hospitals. Our exceptional sepsis survival results and our pressure ulcer results are only due in part to our teams practicing their roles. Practicing generally makes teams better.

One very useful way that we practice various aspects of care delivery is to use robot patients. That work fascinates me. I have written a couple of letters about our robot patients. We use them in multiple settings, and we believe they help us deliver better care. The next letter was the first one I wrote on that topic. More recently, we actually flew two of our robots to Bangladesh to serve as core teaching tools for a school of nursing there. The nursing school in Bangladesh loved the gift. We sent trainers along to show the teachers how to use the robots as teaching tools. So we have come a fairly long way in the use of robots since I wrote this first weekly letter celebrating "patient simulations."

Celebrating Patient Simulator Training – February 15, 2008

Dear KP Colleagues,

Five to ten years from now, health care workers all across the planet will do a significant part of their training using robots as practice patients rather than people.

Five years ago, that concept was completely unheard of.

Robots are a perfect training approach and tool. A life size doll-like piece of machinery can bleed, have seizures, and give birth — allowing experienced caregivers a chance to practice special skills and giving inexperienced trainees a chance to learn brand new skills and new techniques.

Right now, only a very few care sites are using human-like mechanical mannequins for training purposes. Kaiser Permanente is a leader in that field.

My letter this week celebrates our pioneering efforts in using mechanical patients to train and upgrade the skill levels of Kaiser Permanente caregivers.

We now have the life-sized computerized mannequins in over thirty sites — realistically simulating medical emergencies and medical needs for our health care teams. The approach works really well. Studies have shown that our use of simulator training and rehearsals have measurably reduced birth injuries for our perinatal teams, for example.

One official goal of the program is to use the simulated patients to "help a team of experts become an expert team." The program allows nurses and other caregivers to practice medical skills, decision making processes, and critical thinking abilities without risking the well being of actual patients.

As one practitioner said to me, "No one would ever have a pilot learn to fly an airplane with a plane full of passengers." Most pilots learn today using simulators that fully recreate the experience and issues of actually flying their planes.

Using robot patients for training is a very similar experience. It is an approach that allows the caregivers to experience some highly-challenging and relatively rare patient problems without having a real patient at risk. Pilots in training have those same chances to respond to problematic flight situations on their simulators.

The training programs and computerized robot patients have been used at Kaiser Permanente in labor and delivery, anesthesia, operating rooms, emergency departments, neonatal/pediatrics, intensive care units, med/surg units (for special "Rapid Response Teams"), general and interventional radiology, adult and pediatric procedural sedation, and ambulatory surgery and procedural centers.

The "Sim Man" doll can simulate heart attacks. The "Noelle Mom" robot can have a baby and can even deliver twins. The "Sim Baby" doll can simulate resuscitation emergencies.

The mannequin and robot names give a clue as to their use. "Trauma Man" is a giveaway — as is "Mega Code Kid."

The use of robots for caregiver training is important pioneering work at Kaiser Permanente. It is helping us figure out better ways of training caregivers and better approaches for taking care of patients.

In a few years, the rest of health care will be catching up with our work in this area. I strongly suspect in a few more years, people will say to today's caregivers, "Did you actually practice first on live human patients when you trained as a caregiver? Wasn't that scary? What happened when you made a mistake?"

Times change. Approaches change. We are — in some key areas — leading change.

So that's my celebration for this week — our brand new doll collection and everything that those mechanical patients are teaching us about care.

Be well.

George

* * *

Background Note: We Have Great New Electronic Data Connectivity Tools

Our most important use of electronic care support tools isn't the use of training robots for on-site caregivers. Our most powerful and pervasive use of electronic care support tools results from us having complete electronic medical records for all of our patients and all of our care sites. Our electronic medical records give our doctors and other caregivers real-time data about each patient. The electronic medical records give us great patient data. We have also linked up our internal systems — our laboratory systems, imaging centers, and even our pharmacies are all linked electronically to the EMR and the KP caregiver. Our internal data flows in real time to support care. Those same systems now allow us to be a world leader in electronic connectivity with patients and between caregivers. And all of that data connectivity also allows us to do extensive and important medical research that almost no one else can do.

I have written a number of weekly letters celebrating various aspects of our wonderful new electronic toolkit. We spent about four billion dollars putting all of those tools in place and they have already repaid our investment many times over.

As I have celebrated in a couple of other letters, we not only have our electronic medical records for our caregivers, we also have what we think may be the most user-friendly electronic medical library for our caregivers. Our library has all medical journals, medical textbooks, and over 2,500 best practice protocols available in real time to our caregivers.

Patient connectivity is also a key point of our total agenda. We have several tools focused on connectivity with patients. Our direct internet connectivity with our members through our web tool — kp.org — now has over 100 million uses a year from our members.

The next two letters talk about our connectivity successes. The first one deals with some large scale numbers. The second letter talks about using the new connectivity in a very focused way to help kids with asthma.

The world of care is changing. We need to be highly skilled at connectivity to take full advantage of how good care can be.

Celebrating Our E-Connectivity Numbers – March 16, 2012

Dear KP Colleagues,

Our members visited kp.org more than 104 million times in 2011.

We lead the world in electronic connectivity for health care. Our members can make appointments, get lab results, email their doctors, or learn about our care sites electronically. Members love having all of that convenience related to care delivery.

Two weeks ago, I wrote a letter about our new app for smartphones. KP members who have Android devices or iPhones or BlackBerrys can now use those mobile operating systems to get access to their medical records, lab results, and access all of the wonderful connectivity of kp.org.

In the first month after it was released, the new smartphone app was used by our members one million times. A million times is a lot. Convenience is obviously extremely important to a lot of people.

I personally love our connectivity tools.

I stopped off at my care site on the way to work a couple of weeks ago and had my blood drawn — by a wonderfully skillful phlebotomist, I am happy to say.

The blood she drew went off to the lab and I had the first lab results back on my iPhone by 11:00 that morning.

The rest of the tests were completed by that afternoon. And then I had an email conversation with my doctor that same afternoon about the results.

For the rest of the health care world, that kind of connectivity with your doctor and that kind of access to lab results would be called "concierge medicine." It is a rare level of service, and people have to pay a lot of money to a "concierge doctor" to get that level of care. For us, it's normal, everyday care for everybody.

Last year, we had more than 29 million lab results viewed online. We also had more than 12 million e-visits between our patients and our physicians, all giving our patients the same kinds of dialogue, connection, and information-sharing I had with my doctor.

When I tell that story to people outside of KP, they say — "Well, sure, you work at KP. So you can get that kind of electronic connectivity with your doctor and your data. That is clearly special treatment because of your job."

It is special treatment, but we did that same special treatment for our members 12 million special times last year. It wasn't special just for me. It was special for all of us — everyone who is a member and a patient at Kaiser Permanente gets that same special attention.

Convenience is a major goal for us. Making the right thing easy to do is our plan and our strategy and our commitment. That's why 2.5 million of our members simply made their clinic appointments online last year — and close to 10 million times our KP members refilled prescriptions online.

We want patients to refill prescriptions.

Our research and our experience as a provider of care both show us that our patients are a lot more likely to refill and to adhere to their prescriptions when our patients can order refills online and have prescriptions mailed to their home. Care is better and lives are better when convenience happens.

We do the mail-order work really well. J.D. Power and Associates ranked mail-order pharmacies in the country and we were part of that study.

How well did we do?

For the third straight year, we ranked highest in customer satisfaction with mail-order pharmacies in America.

That's a great ranking.

So my letter this week celebrates our connectivity — of all the people who built and operate kp.org — and all of our caregivers who did those much appreciated 12 million e-visits with our patients just last year.

I am also celebrating the Kaiser Permanente mail-order pharmacy team who ranked number one in the entire country for the third straight year.

Nice when that happens.

All very well done.

Be well.

George

☆ ☆ ☆

Celebrating Voice Recognition Calls as Reminders for Kids With Asthma March 9, 2012

Dear KP Colleagues,

Asthma is the fastest growing medical problem for kids in this country.

More kids die of asthma than die from any other chronic condition.

Asthma attacks can be extremely painful and sometimes asthma attacks can kill. One of my own sons had horrible childhood asthma. We spent a lot of time in the emergency room keeping him alive. In the worst year — a couple of decades ago — we spent 27 nights in the ER.

An ER is not a fun place to be with a preteen child and with all of the other patients who come for care after midnight. It's a wonderful place to be when the medications take effect and your son starts breathing normally again — crisis over.

So childhood asthma has a special place on my own list of things to do well.

We do a lot of things really well with asthma care at Kaiser Permanente. My son would have been in the ER a lot less back then if he had the support we give asthma patients now.

We deliver great care to our kid patients with asthma, and we are constantly looking for ways to make that care better.

One of our ways to make asthma care better was just presented at the American Academy of Allergy, Asthma and Immunology 2012 Annual Meeting ⬀.

Our focus as a learning care system was to figure out ways of helping kids with asthma to be equipped with the right medications and to help those patients remember to take their medications.

Because kids are involved, we tested voice recognition-enabled robo calls to remind kids to refill prescriptions and take their medications.

We set up the computer-automated robo calls to help remind the kids and their families to follow their doctors' advice and their treatment plans.

We also added to the call process a live call from a pediatric nurse who specialized in asthma care — having the asthma nurse specialist make a live call if the child's prescriptions were not refilled after the second robo call. And then — to make the right thing easy to do — we tied the calls to our award-winning mail-order pharmacy system. The program was a collaborative effort involving physicians, nurses, pharmacists, and care-givers all working together to improve care.

So what happened?

It turned out to be a very good thing to do.

The robo calls worked. We targeted the robo calls to prescription refills. Far too many kids with asthma do not refill their prescriptions and many suffer crisis events as a result. When that happens, those kids and their parents end up where my son and I used to be — in the emergency room trying to restore breathing to a kid in crisis.

So how well did the calls work?

A study was set up with a control group and a group of kids who got the robo calls.

The group that was called had an average of 52 days between refills. The control group that received no calls averaged 78 days between refills.

The kids in the group who were called were clearly more likely to refill their medications.

The world is changing. Another study presented at that same meet-ing of the Academy of Allergy, Asthma, and Immunology looked at con-nectivity with kids who received text messages about their asthma.

Of the kids with asthma who were sent randomly scheduled text messages about their need for medication adherence, 93 percent believed it improved their care.

Kids like text messages. They tend to live in a world full of text mes-sages. Text messages from their caregivers were well received and gave the care team a great way of targeting messages right to those kids about their asthma care. That approach was also a success.

We are on a path of exploration, trying to figure out ways we can use robo calls, other connectivity tools, and our advanced internal computer-ized database about our patients to make care better. The next generation of great care will involve a whole new set of connectivity strategies and tools that didn't even exist a short while ago. Because we are responsible for the health of close to nine million people, we have a wonderful oppor-tunity to figure out a whole new set of care support tools and approaches — and care will be better as we go through that learning process.

If you would have said to someone a couple of years ago that care delivery would be using text messages and speech recognition-triggered robo calls to support care, whoever you said that to would not have even understood the key words in that sentence. Today, that agenda makes sense.

The future is beginning now.

We are in a great position to help determine how that future will be set up.

We have a lot of very smart people doing very smart, creative, and innovative things that will help define the future of care.

Text messaging is going to be part of our future. So will e-mails, e-education, e-counseling, and e-learning.

We need to figure out how to do all of the new connectivity approaches safely and intelligently and well.

So my letter this week celebrates the researchers in innovation who are working to figure out better ways to deliver asthma care at Kaiser Permanente — and who are looking at future tools to make them realities for us and our patients today.

We published the research because we are helping the world learn, as well.

Well done.

Be well.

George

✿ ✿ ✿

Background Note: Our Members Now Can Get Their Medical Record and Email Their Doctor on Their iPhone, Android or other Smartphone

Way back in early 2011, when I wrote my first weekly letter about our next generation of patient-focused connectivity tools, people had to go to their computers and get on the internet in order to get their lab results, email their doctors, refill their prescriptions, or schedule an appointment with their KP care giver. Those were the clunky olden days. You could connect with us as a patient at multiple levels in 2011 — but some of the best connections required an actual computer.

We are more nimble in our connection links now.

Today, we have managed to extend all of that lovely and convenient connectivity to the smartphone. Androids, iPhones, and other smartphones now directly connect our members with their data and with their caregivers anywhere on the planet. The next letter celebrates that great connectivity leap forward. We may be the only care sites anywhere near our scope and scale who can offer all of those connections to patients everywhere.

Patients love the links. I was just at a meeting in Washington, D.C., where the first speaker held up her iPhone and told the room that she was a Kaiser Permanente member, and she had refilled her prescriptions at 6:30 that morning on her iPhone.

People in the audience who were not Kaiser Permanente members seemed surprised. People in the room who were Kaiser Permanent members agreed that the new connectivity works really well.

Celebrating Our First App – August 19, 2011

Dear KP Colleagues,

We now have an iPhone app.

It is the tip of an iceberg...the next connectivity path on a journey that is turning into a superhighway of connectivity over time.

This is a good path to be on. Americans and the whole world now connect regularly with phone technology none of us could ever have anticipated just a few years ago.

Now we have amazing cell phones and we have a whole range of constantly improving connectivity devices that link people in many ways. There are now so many potentially fun and useful tools and applications for those devices that no one can even count how many available apps there are. The app stores are full of programs to use. People today find restaurants, shop, sell things, keep up friendships, learn, study, teach, get the news, create news, store stuff, share stuff, and connect in a growing number of ways through those various applications.

That's obviously a world Kaiser Permanente needs to be part of.

We need to ride that wave. We need to use those tools and make multiple kinds of connections with our members and patients using those tools.

We are an IT leader already in other areas.

We lead the world today in the use of electronic medical records. No other private health care system in the world comes anywhere near our scope or size for our electronic medical information. We already have real-time medical information about each patient in the exam room and hospital for each patient. Our system for labs, imaging, pharmacy, and care delivery all link with each other today. We basically lead the world in e-visits, secure messaging between patients and physicians, and electronic reporting of test results and lab findings.

Our members signed on to use those functions over sixty-two million times last year.

Our total kp.org website will exceed 70,000,000 total connections with our members this year, including all of the health education, appointment scheduling, and information-sharing functions that our members like to use.

I personally love the ability to have an email dialogue with my doctor. I find that her next ability to reach out electronically with an e-note to remind me when I haven't done follow-up that I need to do is both motivational and care enhancing. It turns out that a mild email and direct reminder note from my doctor can get me both to remember that I need to do tests and then to actually do them. In other care settings, only the people who pay a lot more money to get what they call "concierge medicine" have that kind of linkage with their doctor. We have nearly thirty million connections a year that could require a face-to-face doctor visit in less well-equipped care settings. We actually go past "concierge" medicine in many ways because those solitary practice concierge doctor encounters usually only have limited and incomplete information about their patients. They usually don't have an EMR, so they don't have all the data KP physicians have.

My care is better and I am a better patient because we now have that link that actually reaches into my phone email. I can now read notes on my telephone from my doctor on an airplane.

"Care in the air" is now real at KP.

We can all also get our personal medical record online through My Health Manager.

Other organizations are trying hard to figure out some way of getting some kind of personal health information electronically to their patients. We trump that whole process by going right to the electronic source document and giving our members and our patients EMR-based data. Our members can use the information to get that data anywhere in the world. We can be in Kenya or Belgium or Beijing as a KP member and get on the web and get important personal health information. That is very cool and useful.

So we already lead pretty much everyone in the world in both electronic support for care and in care connectivity at KP. Now we are taking another big step.

What I am celebrating this week is our first actual application for the iPhone. We now have an "app." A real iPhone app.

The app is pretty cool. And useful. What does it do? It helps us find care. You can find it in the iTunes store.

The app supports finding care by specialty with maps and addresses and chances to make choices. Any KP member with an iPhone connection can use the app to find KP care.

We will, of course, reach beyond the iPhone as a linking tool.

We will also build similar apps for other connection devices. We started with an iPhone app and with finding care as a service because we need to start somewhere and that's both a good infrastructure and a good topic to work with. It is the beginning. We will build a whole additional set of apps over the next few years.

In fact, if you have a good idea for a KP app, send it to me and I will pass it on to our app support team.

For now — for this week — I would like to congratulate the team of systems folks and caregivers who did app number one and made it real.

It's well done. It works well. It looks good. And it gives us a presence in a whole new area that is clearly linked to the future of care.

Well done.

Be well.

George

✣ ✣ ✣

Background Note: We Won Several Connectivity Awards at the National Health Care Systems Conference

The next letter briefly mentions our new smartphone app again — but the letter is really celebrating the fact that Kaiser Permanente won a ton of awards for our care computerization and for our total connectivity at the annual Healthcare Information and Management Systems Society (HIMSS) meeting this year.

What awards did we win?

HIMSS rated hospitals across the country for the use of computers. There are more than 5,000 licensed hospitals in the country. Only 66 of those hospitals were rated by HIMSS as being fully computerized, stage 7 hospitals. Thirty-six of those stage 7 hospitals were Kaiser Permanente hospitals.

We swept the hospital computerization awards. We also received the Davies Award for computerization of health care delivery. The next letter celebrates our HIMSS recognitions. Thirty-five thousand health care IT people from all over the world attended that HIMSS conference. It was good to be recognized by those folks, because those are the folks who are moving health care to the next level of system supported performance.

Celebrating KP Recognitions at the Annual HIMSS Conference This Week – February 24, 2012

Dear KP Colleagues,

How many times did our new smartphone access tool get used in the very first month after we made it available to our members and patients?

A million times.

We hit a million uses in one month.

A million is a big number. People really like going to their iPhone or their Android or their Blackberry and getting their lab results, scheduling an appointment, refilling a prescription, or emailing their doctor.

Thirty-five thousand is another big number. This week, there have been 35,000 health care IT people gathered from all over the world to share information about health care IT. This is HIMSS Week. HIMSS Week is a special annual conference for people who love and create health care IT.

"HIMSS" stands for the Healthcare Information and Management Systems Society.

This is the 12th HIMSS annual conference.

HIMSS has speakers, systems demonstrations, a vendor show floor with over 1,000 vendor displays, and a series of awards that are given out every year for health care IT excellence.

One of the HIMSS awards is the Stage 7 Hospital Award. There are more than 5,000 hospitals in the United States. HIMSS rates hospitals on a score of zero to seven on how well the hospitals have computerized their operations.

Only 66 hospitals in the entire country have received the highest Stage 7 Award.

So how did we do?

Thirty-six of the Stage 7 hospitals are us. No one else comes close to KP hospital success levels. We received our 36th Stage 7 Award this week.

The most visible awards at HIMSS are the Davies Awards. HIMSS gives their Davies Awards out every year to the health care organizations that do the best job of using computers to support care.

So who won the Davies Award for Organizational Excellence this year?

We did. All 35,000 people who were gathered at HIMSS learned from the communications for the event that the selection committee for HIMSS presented that award this year to Kaiser Permanente. It's kind of a Health IT Oscar. The Davies trophy is a lot bigger and shinier than an Oscar.

Those awards were not our only HIMSS visibility. We actually were featured and spotlighted a dozen times at separate HIMSS sessions.

Maybe the most newsworthy spotlight session was focused on our joint Care Connectivity Consortium(SM) (CCC) announcement — with a session that was co-led by KP, the Mayo Clinic, and Intermountain Healthcare.

You may remember that Kaiser Permanente and a few of the other best care systems in American health care decided together early last year to collectively figure out a safe and secure way to transfer patient data between care systems when physicians and care teams need that data to help patients.

Electronic health records are wonderful, but they have too often not been able to communicate information well between different sets of electronic records and different care sites. The five CCC founding organizations — Mayo Clinic, Geisinger, Kaiser Permanente, Intermountain Healthcare, and Group Health — all wanted to help create a tool that would safely and securely do that work.

We succeeded. Very smart physician leaders and great system designers and researchers for Kaiser Permanente and the other care systems have managed — in less than one year — to build and use a prototype data connector to do that work. We have actually done our first successful linkages.

It is an amazing breakthrough. The head of HIMSS personally presided over the announcement session when KP, the Mayo Clinic, and Intermountain presented and described our collective success levels to the HIMSS world.

The Care Connectivity Consortium is just beginning its work — but the good news is that it looks as if that work has a high likelihood of success. The entire health care world needs that tool. We are helping to build that tool because it needs to be built.

So it has been a good week for Kaiser Permanente at HIMSS. My letter this week celebrates all of our hospitals who have done a spectacular job of achieving Stage 7 status.

I am also celebrating all of the people who have gotten us to the position where HIMSS believes the Davies Award for Organizational Excellence should be given to us. And I am celebrating the KP teams who did all of the work that has made the CCC collaborative a winner, as well.

Wonderful work.

Well done.

Be well.

George

✿ ✿ ✿

Background Note: The Care Connectivity Consortium is Doing Important Connectivity Work Between the EMR's of World-Class Care Systems

We may well lead the world on internal electronic connectivity. We connect really well inside KP. But external electronic connectivity between care sites is still a huge problem for the rest of the country. One of the challenges for all of health care right now is that many care sites in this country currently have moved from paper files to electronic medical records — but the electronic medical records are usually functionally segregated and simply do not share data or connect with each other.

Splintered and segregated electronic data is just as dysfunctional for patient care as splintered and segregated paper data. We figured that out years ago as a pioneer in the actual functional use of electronic medical data to support care for our own patients, so we have begun to do some work to help various electronic medical records in other care sites connect with each other.

The next two letters celebrate our work in those areas. The first letter celebrates the creation of the Care Connectivity Consortium (CCC) — a joint effort among Kaiser Permanente and four of the best care organizations in America to create a working electronic connectivity tool. The Mayo Clinic, Geisinger Health System, Intermountain Health Care, and Group Health Cooperative of Puget Sound are the cofounders of the new Care Connectivity Consortium with us. That effort is already bearing fruit. As of today, all five sites are actually successfully achieving data connectivity for individual patients.

That is huge progress for great care systems in a relatively short time.

The second letter celebrates an earlier effort between Kaiser Permanente and the Veterans Administration to do very similar work. That pioneering work with the VA has been a lovely starting point, and it was an important learning foundation for the CCC work. I have celebrated both of those efforts with more than one weekly letter. These two tell the story.

Celebrating the Care Connectivity Consortium – April 8, 2011

Dear KP Colleagues,

The headline in the New York Times said — "Big Medical Groups Begin Patient Data-Sharing Project."

They were writing about us. Us and four other world-class medical groups.

We have formed a consortium with the Mayo Clinic, the Geisinger Health System, Intermountain Healthcare, and Group Health Cooperative of Seattle to create a process and a system for linking data between electronic medical records.

The medical groups in the consortium all are EMR pioneers. Kaiser Permanente has the private-health-care-world's largest and most complete EMR — but the other members of the new consortium also have millions of patients in their electronic medical records.

We are all using our EMRs to improve care and support the delivery of care. We are all learning how to use that wonderful new tool — and we are all interested in sharing what we are learning with the world.

In the old days, all medical information was locked into paper medical files. The paper records were isolated in file drawers — and if a patient had five physicians providing care, the data was generally locked into five separate and isolated filing cabinets in five different care settings.

Electronic records are much better than paper records. Electronic records are accessible, intelligible, and much more accurate than paper records. Electronic records can link with one another — so all of the data for a patient can be available in real time in a single access process.

Electronic is better.

The problem with electronic is that when patients go to different doctors for their care, they still tend to have separate records — and that can create electronic silos instead of paper silos.

That isn't a problem inside Kaiser Permanente for the vast majority of our patients because our physicians can generally share patient medical records. But it is a problem in other settings, and it can be a challenge for us when patients go outside our system for some of their care.

That problem is an even bigger challenge for the other members of our new consortium — because they have a higher percentage of their patients getting at least some of their care from other sites.

In a perfect world, all of the care sites would be connected, and in a perfect world the data would flow with the patient from site to site.

We want a perfect world — so we are now working to create the kind of computer-to-computer data flows that will allow that piece of perfection to happen, safely and securely.

We piloted a connection like that with the Veterans Administration — linking the two largest electronic medical records in the country. Those linkages worked.

So we are now committed to creating similar linkages with the new set of elite medical groups to create a process that works first for our patients and then — if we do it well — for the world.

It's a real solid set of fellow pioneers. The leaders of each of the five care systems held a press conference in Washington, D.C., at the National Press Club on Wednesday of this week. You can link to the press conference here. We had two presenters at the conference. A copy of the press release for the conference is available on our News Center.

We are being saluted by key leaders in Washington for our efforts.

This is important work. If someone doesn't figure out how to create links between electronic medical records, those records will not be linked.

It will not be done until someone does it.

Who better than us to do it?

We are patient-focused and we know what can be done and we know what should be done with an EMR.

Almost all other care sites are just getting their toes in the water. Some are getting their feet wet. We are swimming.

So this is a good contribution for us to make. Instead of keeping our advances and our learning secret and special only to us, we are sharing what we know because we want care to be better for everyone.

Sharing is good.

So my letter this week celebrates all of the people on our care delivery team and our IT team who have been working hard to get this new Care Connectivity Consortium℠ up and running.

Good work.

Well done.

Be well.

George

✭ ✭ ✭

Celebrating EMR Connectivity – October 3, 2008

Dear KP Colleagues,

Most of health care uses paper medical records to keep track of the care that is delivered to individual patients.

The paper records are generally locked into separate file cabinets, in separate rooms and separate buildings — relatively inaccessible, completely unlinked with each other, often incomplete, sometimes inaccurate, sometimes illegible, and almost always totally inert. The information about care locked in those paper files is a rich array of data that doesn't do anywhere near as much good as it could and should do for patients.

In contrast, with KP HealthConnect® we have led the world in putting together an electronic medical record that makes all of the information about all of the patients available all of the time.

Other caregivers in several settings have also implemented electronic medical records — but in contrast to our data set, those records tend to be relatively incomplete — often containing only the hospital-based care from a single hospital or the specialty-based care from a single specialty group for their patients. We are both a health plan and a "vertically integrated" total care system, but the other folks with electronic medical records tend to be stand-alone care delivery sites, so their data tends to be very site specific — not patient focused.

We are far from perfect in our electronic medical record agenda, but we are moving in some pretty good directions at a pretty good pace.

Most people in health care policy circles applaud what we are doing and have done. But some folks in Washington have had a major worry. Their concern is that even though electronic medical records are obviously far superior to paper records, it may be possible that the new EMR data sets that are being built will, in the end, just create new site-specific silos of unconnected electronic data. They worry that even though Kaiser Permanente is building a great EMR agenda, and even though other organizations like The Mayo Clinic, Geisinger Clinic, Cleveland Clinic, and the Veterans Administration (VA) are all building next generation EMRs — we may now be on a path as a country to create segregated electronic data sets for each of those caregivers.

Some people in Washington are so concerned about that possibility of unlinkable electronic data that they have proposed that Congress should now dictate a single medical record format and system to be used by all caregivers. They salute us for the progress we have made, but wonder if we should be using some standardized federal medical record system rather than KP HealthConnect.

We heard that concern. So we decided to do something important and useful in response. We went to the Veterans Administration — the other most successful EMR in America — and we put together a project with the VA to see if we could get our EMR to talk to their EMR.

We had some very smart people from Kaiser Permanente and the VA get together to figure out if the two systems could communicate with each other for the care of a given patient — kind of like the way banks communicate with each other relative to cash machines and data flow.

What I am celebrating this week is the success of that pilot process. At a meeting last week in Washington, D.C., in front of the Secretary of the Department of HHS and hundreds of Congressional Staffers, we and senior officials from the VA showed how the data flow could be linked so that a patient from the VA could be served in multiple VA settings, then in various Kaiser Permanente settings, and then back in the VA — with care data available at every site of care.

The project was a major success. It showed that those linkages were, in fact, possible. The pilot project along with a few others of a similar nature, pointed Washington toward a national agenda of connectivity rather than a national strategy of perfect system conformity.

Local television stations ran stories about the press conference. Online media also covered the story.

Most importantly, policy people working on those issues in health care IT policy circles now know another solution is possible.

About half way through the project, we heard from Washington that the government had run out of money in that particular budget and could not complete the work. We had two choices — kill the project, or help them fund their share. We opted to help them fund their side of the project because we believed so strongly that America needed to know whether this connectivity approach could work.

So my congratulations this week are both to the people on our team who made the project a success and the people on our team who had the creativity and initiative to figure out how to get the project to the finish line even though the government budget was killed. It took nearly a million dollars on our part, but a key point in the total health reform strategy for our country was at risk — so we decided to help make the connectivity effort a learning process and a win.

So, thank you team.

Be well.

George

✱ ✱ ✱

Background Note: Electronic Data Tees Up and Supports Great, Valuable, and Invaluable Research

I love health care research. I love it when we learn something new that saves lives and improves care.

Our new electronic data tools help us improve care, and they also allow us to do some great research. We have always done great research at Kaiser Permanente — and we are able to do even better research now with the new data flow.

Quite a few of my weekly letters deal with our research learnings and wins.

Most people have no idea how extensive the Kaiser Permanente research agenda is.

Kaiser Permanente does roughly 1,000 research projects every year. We have one of the largest research agendas of any care system on the planet. We learn a lot, and we share our learnings with the world by publicizing our research.

Now, we are on a path to do even better research in some key areas. We now have a lovely database and we have more than nine million patients who tend to be with us over extended periods of time, so we have an incredible opportunity to do some very meaningful research about time-based care development and care impacts.

The next couple of celebration letters shared some of our research wins and talked about our research agendas and goals with our staff.

Celebrating KP Research as a Gift to the World – December 23, 2011

Dear KP Colleagues,

Our research really is a gift to the world.

We have a lovely research agenda at KP. We have an almost perfect research environment. We have patients. Our patients stay with us for a very long time.

A lot of research environments scramble for a tiny set of patients. We have millions of possible research-linked patients.

We provide all of the care for most of our patients. Most research settings only provide a piece of the patient's care.

We have electronic medical records instead of paper medical records. The advantages of electronic records when it comes to research abilities are spectacular. We don't have to hunt through file cabinets full of splintered paper records to do our learning.

We do our research for the right reasons.

We want to do research to make the world a better place.

Many other research teams are targeted at cash returns, profits, and generating corporate wealth.

We are aimed at knowledge, not wealth; and our research is targeted at intellectual expansion and better care, not financial growth.

It isn't sinful to do research to generate financial gain — but it is a very good thing not to be limited, constrained, or focused by that agenda.

We do research to figure out ways we can make care better for our patients and for the world.

We have a great team of researchers. We have great systems. We have a great database. We have a magnificently diverse patient population. We are very careful to protect patient confidentiality — and we have the right processes in place to get the right approvals when approvals are part of the process.

We have a great set of values and we have the right set of motivations.

And — as a result of that mix of good things — we are doing some very nice research.

This week we published a research paper showing that early intervention with pregnant women at risk of substance abuse has an extremely good outcome for mothers and children. We showed that early and consistent screening and basic early interventions can make care a lot better for mothers and children — and we are even able to say that if the entire country adopted our approach and used our screening interventions, the country could save about $2 billion on care costs for those families.

Our study involved 49,000 pregnant women in our KP care system. That research was done as part of a major operational attempt to create better care. It was practical work done by practical and caring people because those situations involving substance abuse can damage lives — and we want to help reduce the levels of that damage.

We succeeded. Now we are sharing what we learned.

A couple of weeks ago, we released another important study that showed the use of ACE inhibitors did not create birth defects.

For that study, we looked at more than 465,000 births.

Earlier research in other settings warned that ACE inhibitor medication might increase birth defects. Women who needed the ACE inhibitors for their hypertension were being warned not to take drugs they needed for their own care.

That can create a real problem for mothers who need their hypertension under control.

Our research made a huge contribution because we were able to look at a large population over a long time and say — that link does not appear to be true.

Sometimes it's important to find a link. Sometimes it is equally important to show that a link doesn't exist.

Hardly anybody other than us has the kind of data size, scope, and availability to do that kind of de-linking research.

It's a blessing and a gift.

We also released important research this month showing that a link does exist between diabetes, depression, and dementia.

Diabetics who suffer from depression have a double risk of developing dementia five years after the initial depression diagnosis. The risk was significantly greater than the risk of dementia for people who were either diabetic or depressed.

Roughly, 20 percent of our patients with diabetes also suffer from depression. We now have good reason to be particularly focused on the patients with both conditions.

The list of effective and needed KP research findings is a large one. We just did a great study showing that kids with diabetes have a higher risk of asthma, and kids with both conditions have a much tougher time keeping their blood sugar under control.

That is the kind of research that is needed for the new computerized care support tools that will be helping the next generation of caregivers figure out where to focus their attention for each individual patient.

We did another study that ran in over 300 media outlets — including USA Today, ABC News, CBS News, and Forbes — that explained that there was not a link between ADHD medications and serious cardiovascular events. That study was another de-linking home run.

At the other end of the continuum, we released a study showing a significant link existed between magnetic field exposure during pregnancy and subsequent asthma in kids. Media around the world also ran articles about that research.

More than 400 news media outlets ran articles about our highly useful research showing a link between medication taken during pregnancy and autism in kids. We have done a number of studies about autism that are becoming important to the world medical information base about the causes of that rapidly growing disease.

Overall, this year alone, we did more than 1,000 separate research projects and we published almost 700 peer-reviewed professional journal articles and counting.

We do very nice research. And care is better because we do it.

So my letter this week celebrates all of our researchers... celebrating our caregivers and care teams who do research and celebrating all of the people who do the systems support and the care analysis that makes our research solid and useful and a gift to the world.

Care literally is better and health care is smarter because our research happens. It's a very good thing to be giving gifts. We do it over and over again because it's the right thing to do and because we actually can make those gifts happen.

Have a great holiday season.

Be well.

George

* * *

Background Note: Autism is One of Our Research Targets

We publish hundreds of research articles every year, so I have a lot of great research fodder to work with for my weekly letters. Much of the research that I write about in my weekly letters deals with major population health issues like autism or Alzheimer's disease — areas where our unique ability to look back into people's prior medical history can create insights that generally may not be available to medical researchers in any other research format or setting.

We discovered, for example, that when pregnant women take a particular drug early in their pregnancy, the risk of autism triples in their kids. That research required a multi-layer database — with longitudinal and complete information about both mothers and children over years. We also discovered that older fathers — fathers over 40 — created a much higher level of autism risk than older mothers. Other research has since validated our findings about older dads and autism risks.

We are looking for those kinds of connections so that we can help reduce the explosion in new autism cases.

Autism is one of the areas where we are looking hard at connectivity linkages — trying to figure out why autism cases have been doubling in this country.

The next letter celebrates some of that research, and also talks about work we are doing to explain why the number of childhood asthma cases are also growing.

Celebrating Finding Underlying Causes and Hidden Connections for Autism – July 15, 2011

Dear KP Colleagues,

The number of kids with autism is growing rapidly.

No one knows why.

There is a lot of speculation. Some people believe that the problem is genetic. Others believe it is environmental.

Most people who study the problem think that some combination of genetic, environmental, and prenatal factors are causing the increases.

Kids with autism can end up with a very challenging life. Parents and families of autistic kids can end up having their own lives redefined and refocused by the needs of their children.

It's a real problem — so any work that can be done to help figure out why kids have autism is extremely important.

We just did some of that work. We took a look into the KP database and looked at some issues relating to prenatal issues for mothers. We just did an important study showing that the risk of autism doubled in children whose mothers took certain drugs during pregnancy. Our researchers also found that the risk of autism tripled for children when mothers took those drugs in the first trimester of pregnancy.

The overall number of children who were exposed to those drugs in utero is pretty low — so the doubled risk was not a large number of births — but the major increase in risk of autism from a prenatal influence was a very important finding to discover.

Some other new research — done by us in collaboration with other researchers outside of KP also announced this month — looked at twins and autism rates. That study concluded that autism could not be entirely genetic, because identical twins had different rates of autism. Some other factors had to be involved. We now know that one of those factors for some of the kids might be the prescribed medications taken by the mothers.

We have been doing a lot of work aimed at discovering the causes of autism. We studied, for example, whether kids who were exposed to antenatal ultrasound in the womb were more likely to be autistic. Our data showed that those children were not more likely to have autism.

That was good to learn, because some people feared that the increasing number of ultrasounds being done were causing an increase in autism.

We also looked at whether exposure in the womb to anti-D immune globulin — medicine used to prevent a potentially serious immunological condition known as Rhesus disease — had a statistical link to autism.

The good news was it did not have that link.

We looked at whether certain vaccines given to moms during pregnancy and to their kids in the first two years of life created a risk for autism.

Our data showed that the suspected vaccines also had no link to autism. Many parents have feared that the vaccine link to autism might exist — so the number of kids being vaccinated has been going down in some areas.

That, of course, is dangerous for the kids. We know from other Kaiser Permanente studies that the death rate from whooping cough — or pertussis — has really spiked due to parents not vaccinating kids. Hundreds of kids have died, because the risk of this disease goes up when kids are not vaccinated.

So our research is helpful in several ways. We are learning where risk happens, and we are learning where risk doesn't happen, in multiple areas.

Because we have such a huge database, and because we have data on entire families available electronically to our research teams, we can do connected levels of research that almost no one else can do.

On the recent prescription during pregnancy study, almost no other care team anywhere has equivalent ongoing data for both mothers and their children. So knowing that a mother was taking a particular prescription in the first trimester of a pregnancy would be something that a care site that only had access to data about the actual kids would probably never have.

Anyone else trying to do that important research would need to look into multiple separate and siloed data files for each of the mothers, and then try to find the equivalent level of data in multiple other separated sites for each of the kids. Their research would be highly incomplete, difficult to assemble, and very expensive to do.

We have great family level data. It is on the computer. The important link we found last year between amniotic fluid infections during pregnancy and childhood asthma could probably not have been done in almost any other care site in the world.

We are blessed with a great data resource. We owe it to the world to keep using our data gold mine to improve the science of health care for everyone.

Autism will continue to be a target for that research. We learned and taught two years ago that the risk of autism increased by about thirty percent if the mother was over forty — and it increased by about fifty percent if the father was over forty.

Some people suspected that the risk of having autistic kids increased with the age of the mother. Few people suspected that the risk also increased with the age of the father.

Again — that kind of research takes large populations of patient data, and it takes stability of the data over time.

More than 700 newspapers, news magazines, TV stations, and radio outlets including the Wall Street Journal, TIME, ABC World News, CBS News, and NPR ran stories about our most recent autism study.

My letter this week celebrates our researchers who are working hard and hitting home runs on our collective quest to figure out the important scientific connections that will save lives and improve lives.

Well done.

Be well.

George

☆ ☆ ☆

Background Note: We Can Use Really Big Data Sets to Save Lives with Research

As I said, I love our research.

A couple of dozen of my weekly letters over the past five years have celebrated various specific research findings published by our Kaiser Permanente research teams. As I noted earlier, we actually have one of the largest research programs of any non-academic care organization in the world. We do a lot more research than a great number of academic institutions and we also train roughly a thousand medical residents in various specialties every year — so we are definitely not non-academic. But as a pure research site, we are huge. Some of the research we do is solid, very basic, fundamental and traditional medical research that could be done anywhere care is delivered. And some of our population-based research is highly dependent on our new electronic medical record database. That array of research efforts would be very hard to do in any other setting.

The next two letters are in that category. Both of the letters talk about some of our special attributes we have as a research center because we have such great support from a huge and growing database of electronic data from our computerized medical records.

The research project addresses the health of kids. The second letter deals with incredibly important information we have learned that can cut deaths from stroke by half for hospitalized patients.

We looked at every single stroke victim in a large population for several entire years to figure out how to save those lives.

I also love our data resource. Care is better and lives are being saved because we have that computerized information and because we can make care better in a systematic way when we learn important new things.

The rest of the world is trying to figure out how to use what we have learned about reducing stroke deaths. We are using that information today.

Celebrating Helping the World Use Our Health Care Data – August 13, 2010

Dear KP Colleagues,

Who in the world other than us can do an important medical study on 700,000 kids and do it without anyone needing to leave our research center?

We just did a study showing the relationship between extreme obesity and gastroesophageal reflux disease (GERD) in extremely obese kids.

GERD is a painful disease. Stomach fluid backs up into people's throats. The disease causes pain and can cause real damage over time. It is also tied to cancer of the esophagus.

That is now the fastest growing cancer in the United States.

People have been wondering if the explosion in obesity and the growing levels of that cancer might be related. Our study shows that GERD and obesity are strongly linked in kids... and that information is helping medical scientists think through the full sets of relationships that might exist.

This was a huge study. It was published in the International Journal of Pediatric Obesity and then more than 100 news outlets ran stories about the research, including CNN Health.com, WebMD, and U.S. News & World Report.

We could do the study of all of those kids because we have our electronic medical records — and our secure records allow us to pull medical information about millions of kids to do important research while protecting their privacy.

We know what their diagnoses are. We know what their treatments are. We know their height and weight and age. We know a ton of data points that can allow real research to happen.

Doing that study would have been incredibly difficult without our new tool kit.

Imagine having only paper medical records with the records for 700,000 kids scattered among tens of thousands of unconnected caregivers. Trained researchers would have had to go to each of those medical offices to sort through all of those individual paper files looking for the right diagnosis language for each of the kids.

They would also have needed to write down in logs the relevant weights for those 700,000 kids at each of their weigh-ins over the past two years. Paper files are not transportable. The researchers would have had to go to all of the medical offices where the paper files are kept to get each piece of data for each of the 700,000 kids.

It would have been a nightmare. It would have cost millions of dollars and possibly taken years to do that research manually. And then it would have been just a snapshot — and any follow-up research would have required all of those researchers to get back in their cars and return to all of those medical offices to see if they can find and get updated information from more than 700,000 paper files.

That's why so little population research is done anywhere in health care. It's clunky and expensive and slow. And the accuracy levels are always suspect for a paper-based research project.

Why are the accuracy levels suspect? Because people would need to individually read and then interpret each of those 700,000 paper files in order to do that study with paper medical files. Interpretation can be very problematic. And a key question has to be, do the doctors in those thousands of separate offices all use the same terms and the same codes? Who coordinates the relevant definitions for the many thousands of doctors who would have been needed to treat 700,000 kids?

The situation is very different for Kaiser Permanente.

Our database uses one set of codes. Our database uses one set of definitions. When we note something is a particular thing, we have reason to believe we are speaking the same language to one another.

The rest of the world aspires to that status, but it isn't there yet. We are where we are because we made a conscious choice in the interest of optimal medical science to do the research we do. We have an obligation to the world to do this kind of research, because we can.

It's a good place to be. Our GERD research is another step in that process.

WE CAN USE REALLY BIG DATA SETS TO SAVE LIVES WITH RESEARCH

So my letter this week celebrates all of our medical thinkers and researchers who are figuring out how we can help the world understand key issues and achieve optimal health and optimal care.

We haven't yet reached that optimal goal, but we are definitely on that path.

Be well.

George

✼ ✼ ✼

Celebrating Our Stroke Research Saving Lives – June 1, 2012

Dear KP Colleagues,

We just did another very important research study that could change care everywhere and confirm treatment patterns everywhere for one of the most common causes of patient deaths in the world — stroke.

We learned how to cut the death rate of stroke victims who are in the hospital by nearly half — reducing mortality levels of our hospitalized stroke patients from 11 percent to only 6 percent.

We also learned what treatment approach can be used to increase the number of stroke patients who can return to their homes by 21 percent.

Our researchers at the Neuroscience Group at Redwood City Medical Center looked at data from 12,689 ischemic stroke patients from all of our Northern California hospitals over a 7-year period. We have a lovely database and we used that data again to learn something really important about how to improve the delivery of care and save lives.

What did we learn?

Statins work. Statins work even better when used quickly after a stroke patient is hospitalized.

We learned that cholesterol-reducing drugs given to stroke patients in the hospital reduce the death rate for stroke patients by nearly half.

That is a "wow" piece of information. Other care programs have recommended use of statins for post-discharge treatment for stroke patients. We learned that lives can be saved relative to the first stroke if that treatment begins immediately for those patients.

It's a very important piece of learning that no one knew until we figured it out. Our research showed that when ischemic stroke patients were given cholesterol-lowering statins while they were still in the hospital after a stroke, the death rate for those patients was cut almost in half, and the numbers of patients who managed to return to their own homes instead of going to a nursing home actually increased by more than 20 percent.

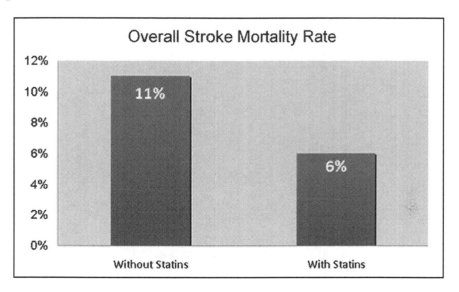

We also learned — and this is also extremely important to know — that if a stroke patient had actually been taking statins before the stroke and we continued that medication in the hospital, the death rate dropped to 5 percent. So keeping a patient on that medication had the very lowest death rate of any approach.

We also learned — at the other extreme — that if the hospitalized stroke patient was already taking statins and if that treatment was stopped at the time of the stroke, the death rate for those patients jumped to 23 percent. So a statins-taking stroke patient who continued taking the medication in the hospital after the stroke had only a 5 percent death rate — a 1 in 20 chance of dying.

But if the statins were discontinued, the death rate jumped to 23 percent — almost 1 in 4 chance of dying.

We are the only people in health care who have done that analysis. Our stroke researchers have done truly great work. This finding has the potential to save many lives.

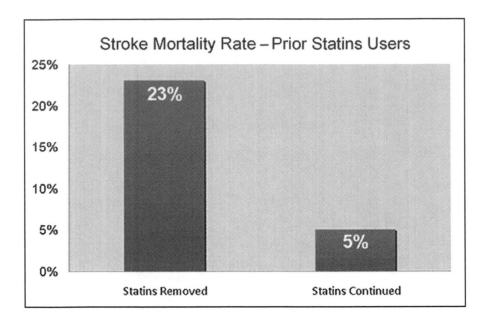

Every stroke-treatment program on the planet Earth can and should either start to give or continue to give cholesterol-lowering statins to their stroke patients. When that happens, lives will be saved.

The research study was published in the peer-reviewed journal, Neurology. A couple of dozen media outlets have run stories about the research.

This finding is another example of why we believe we are on the cusp of a golden age for medical research — because we can now use real data in volume levels to discover things that could never be known or discovered without the data. The researchers in this study applied very sophisticated statistical controls and techniques to give us great confidence in the findings.

Before we did that research, no one knew that those impacts existed during those hospital stays. Our data shows that lives can be saved if we do the right thing for stroke patients in the hospital.

So what are we doing with that new information at Kaiser Permanente?

Our patients are benefitting.

We are using that knowledge to improve care.

We have already added that lovely information from our research scientists to the care delivery practices for our patients. The automated

Kaiser Permanente HealthConnect® "Stroke Order Sets" have now been changed so that high-dose statins therapy starting on day one of care is now the "default order set" for ischemic stroke patients.

The KP National Cardiovascular Disease (CVD) Risk Reduction Guidelines from CMI have been updated to include this new medical wisdom. Our CMI electronic clinical medical Library is sharing this information with our caregivers. We are also providing ongoing physician-to-physician educational opportunities about the new information.

We are a learning organization in the best sense of that term.

So my letter this week celebrates the researchers who did the analysis to figure out that those extremely important linkages exist.

My letter also celebrates the teams who build and upgrade our care protocols and our systems support tools.

And I am celebrating all of the caregivers at Kaiser Permanente who will now use that information to make care better.

This is another key quality win.

We already have what may be the lowest death rates in the country from sepsis. We probably already have the lowest death rates from heart disease. We now could be on a path to have the lowest death rates in the country from stroke.

That is incredibly important work. We are sharing what we have learned with the world. The odds are good that we will be indirectly helping to save lives across a broad expanse of care settings.

That's very much a good thing to do.

Well done, Kaiser Permanente research teams.

And well done, Kaiser Permanente medical record support teams.

Well done, Kaiser Permanente caregivers.

It's good to make a difference.

Be well.
George

* * *

Background Note: Not All of Our Research Uses Electronic Data – Reducing SIDS Deaths, for Example, Was Great Non-Electronic Research

As I have pointed out in multiple letters, we really do a lot of research at Kaiser Permanente — roughly a thousand published papers every year. Some of our most visible research involves use of our total electronic data resource. But that is only a piece of our research work. Much of our research is not related in any way to our medical record. It is pure, old-fashioned research involving traditional observations of patients and processes.

The next letter celebrates an amazing and important piece of research that was done at Kaiser Permanente relative to Sudden Infant Death Syndrome — SIDS. That syndrome has been another area of research focus for us. We have actually achieved a couple of very important insights into SIDS deaths.

This is the kind of research finding that should be available to parents and to caregivers all over the world. The potential reduction in those tragic SIDS deaths could be huge across the entire planet.

The fact that these numbers about how to prevent SIDS are so striking, and yet so few people know that this research has been done is an indictment, all by itself, of how badly our current non-system of care as a country disseminates important scientific information to care givers and patients — and in this case — to parents of patients.

The letter is, however, a celebration — not an indictment.

Celebrating SIDS Research Study - October 24, 2008

Dear KP Colleagues,

Our research team just hit another home run.

Sudden Infant Death Syndrome is one of the saddest diseases in the world. Otherwise healthy children — infants — sometimes simply die, with no medical condition that can be diagnosed that could have caused their death.

It's a major tragedy when a SIDS death occurs. Families often go through pain and grief for a very long time.

Our researchers at Kaiser Permanente have been looking for the cause of those deaths and our researchers have also been looking for ways to prevent those deaths.

That research is paying off. We now have credible research that we believe can significantly reduce the number of SIDS cases.

I suspect none of us could have guessed what the two approaches are that seem to work.

We released a study two years ago showing that the risk of SIDS deaths was reduced by more than 90 percent in babies who used pacifiers.

Our newest study — released two weeks ago — showed a 72 percent reduction in the risk of SIDS deaths for babies who have a fan blowing moving air onto their cribs when they are sleeping. The theory is that the moving air dispels the carbon dioxide buildup that can occur when the expelled breath air isn't moving away from the baby's face.

That is a very important discovery. It deals both with the issue of what may cause SIDS and what can be done to prevent it roughly 72 percent of the time.

The outside world believes that is an important learning. More than 700 media outlets ran the story — including The New York Times, The Wall Street Journal, USA Today, Associated Press, HealthDay and TIME. It was also on television and multiple radio shows, including NBC's "The Today Show," ABC News, CBS News, KQED Radio, KCBS Radio, Voice of America and Ivanhoe National Broadcast News. You can see the research online.

Kaiser Permanente research is saving lives. Our willingness to share that research with the world is one of the reasons why it is having an impact. We don't simply publish our research in a professional journal with a small circulation and hope that someone reads it. We focus on the research that can make a difference in the world, and we make the physicians and other Kaiser Permanente researchers who did the studies available to the news media to help explain exactly why and how the research is important.

We do more than learn. We teach.

So this week I am celebrating both the researchers who did this important work and our team who talked to the world to share the information.

Pediatricians and mothers all over the world will finally have valid advice to give and take on SIDS because of our work.

Be well.

George

✿ ✿ ✿

Background Note: Diabetes, Obesity, and Dementia are Also Areas of Research Focus

The next two letters deal with research done on three of our favorite healthcare topics — diabetes, obesity, and dementia. Each of those conditions develops over time — and each of those conditions is growing in impact relative to our overall population. We are trying very hard to figure out important things about patients in each of those categories.

We can do some great research in those areas.

We have great longitudinal data at Kaiser Permanente — with many patients staying with us over many years. We have the most loyal members of any health plan, measured by annual renewal rates. The fact that we have members staying with us as a care system and a health plan over long periods of time allows us to learn some important things about the progression of health conditions.

The next couple of letters celebrate some of that learning.

Celebrating Kaiser Permanente Research – August 29, 2008

Dear KP Colleagues,

The number of pregnant women with diabetes has doubled in only six years.

That piece of research done by Kaiser Permanente made news all over the world earlier this year — with more than 800 newspapers, magazines, radio stations and TV shows running stories about that particular research project.

Another 500 radio stations, TV news shows, newspapers and magazines did stories about the fact that keeping food diaries was one of the best ways of losing weight.

Several national news shows featured that Kaiser Permanente research-based story. Reporters loved that information. Weight loss is incredibly difficult, and our research showed that food diaries actually made a major difference for a very high percentage of people.

Another extremely important Kaiser Permanente study showed that immediate weight loss after being diagnosed as being diabetic made a major difference in preventing some complications of diabetes for a high percentage of people. That study is very important because it tells medical science that we can, in fact, make a very big difference in the quality of health and life outcomes for new diabetics — to an extent no one thought possible — just by losing weight at that specific time.

That study will become a staple learning tool for diabetic care everywhere. We will continue to distribute it. Over 100 media outlets have featured that story to date.

One of the biggest single media exposures for a Kaiser Permanente research project so far this year was the 1,800 news stories that were run about the link our researchers discovered between mid-life "pot bellies" and late-life dementia. Who knew? No one.

Mid-life "belly fat" turned out to be a disproportionate predictor of certain brain functioning problems later in life.

Only Kaiser Permanente could have done that last study. Why? Because no one else has so many years of data. We have a several decades-old investment in keeping medical data on file — and we have very loyal members and patients who stay with us over long periods of time — so we were able to look back 35 years into a blinded-version of people's medical data base to see the correlation between early belly fat and late dementia.

We don't know anyone else who has that kind of longitudinal data base about care.

As I have said in earlier letters, our new KP HealthConnect® system is designed in part to give us the best research data base in health care. That new system builds on a long and proud Kaiser Permanente tradition of recording data about care and then using the data to do meaningful research about care.

All four of those research projects can be accessed by going to their Web links — listed below.

- ¤ Pre-Pregnancy Diabetes
- ¤ Food Diaries
- ¤ Diabetes and Weight Loss
- ¤ Belly Fat Dementia

I celebrated another set of research projects earlier this year. Since that time, we have released a number of additional studies, and our total 2008 news media story count from our Kaiser Permanente research has now exceeded 6,100 placements, year-to-date.

We are doing important research. We are also sharing it with the world — and we are helping other caregivers and patients learn from our learning.

So that's my celebration this week — thanking and congratulating our research teams who continue to do such exceptional work.

Be well.

George

* * *

Celebrating Our Research Teams – April 17, 2009

Dear KP Colleagues,

Reuters, the international news service, ran a story Wednesday of this week that said:

"Older diabetics whose blood sugar drops to dangerously low levels have a higher risk of developing dementia, U.S. researchers said on Tuesday.

The study by researchers at Kaiser Permanente in Oakland, California, suggests that aggressive blood sugar control resulting in blood sugar so low it requires a trip to the hospital may increase dementia risks in older adults with type 2 diabetes."

The study ran in JAMA and it used more than two decades of Kaiser Permanente data. It basically gave a warning to the health care world that intense hypoglycemia can increase the likelihood of dementia. One episode increases risk by 45 percent. Two episodes increased risk by 115 percent. Three or more episodes ran the risk up 160 percent.

That story also ran Wednesday in three of the most widely read newspapers in America — The New York Times, USA Today, and The Wall Street Journal. It was picked up by more than 200 other media outlets and it was featured on a couple of national television shows.

Again our researchers are learning things that can influence both care and health for people all over the world, and we are sharing that information with the world.

The researchers used our database and the fact that we have loyal, long-standing members, to reach conclusions about long-term health situations that would be hard for almost anyone but us to do.

So I am celebrating our research team and the KP Division of Research for doing really important research. I want to particularly congratulate the Northern California Diabetes Registry Team for years of really solid work that is letting us add this kind of value to the world of medical science.

Alzheimer's is the most common form of dementia in older people. Diabetes is the fastest-growing chronic disease. More than twenty-three million Americans have diabetes.

This is an area where increased learning can make a real difference for a lot of people. Dementia can be a heartbreaking condition. People drift out of control of their own thought processes and lose layers of awareness and functionality. It can be a very sad thing.

So if we can use our research to help people avoid medical situations that increase the risk of dementia by 160 percent, that really is a wonderful thing to do. This is important work. We should be proud of the people on our team who did that work.

So congratulations again to our researchers for a job well done.

Be well.

George

✳ ✳ ✳

Background Note: We Have Also Studied Causes of Sexual Dysfunction

The next letter also addresses a couple of Kaiser Permanente research topics that caught the attention of the media world — the link between cholesterol levels in our 30s and 40s and dementia in later years was one topic. Sexual dysfunction created by high levels of exposure to a specific chemical was another.

Both studies are causing people to think differently about a couple of key health care topics. Those linkages were not known before we detected them. Learning that those linkages existed was also good research to celebrate in a weekly letter.

Celebrating Research into Environmental Consequences - November 13, 2009

Dear KP Colleagues,

Unexpected consequences can make major differences in people's lives. A couple of months ago, I wrote about our Kaiser Permanente research study that showed that being significantly overweight and having very high cholesterol levels in our thirties and forties can increase our personal risk of dementia in our sixties and seventies by roughly 360 percent.

Three hundred and sixty is a big increase in risk.

A lot of other research has shown that weight problems and high cholesterol can definitely increase heart disease, diabetes, stroke, and even cancer. Those negative consequences were known before we did our study.

Our research took that learning a big step further — and the world now knows that excess weight and high cholesterol also significantly increase the risk of Alzheimer's.

Thousands of newspapers, magazines, and media outlets ran that story.

We now have another research study that is generating hundreds of articles and stories this week.

The study released this week is about environmental risk. Our research team identified the fact that high levels of exposure to the chemical bisphenol A (BPA) can lead to significant sexual dysfunction. People have speculated for years that particular chemical might cause problems in humans — and studies on animals have already shown major negative results — but some people who defended the wide use of BPA in making hard plastic bottles and other manufactured goods have said that there were no studies showing similar negative impacts on humans.

That was true until now.

Kaiser Permanente researchers studied male factory workers in China who had high levels of exposure to BPA, and the research results are pretty conclusive.

Damage results from high levels of BPA exposure.

We released those research findings to the world on Tuesday. So far this week, USA Today, Associated Press, ABC News.com, CNN, U.S. News & World Report, HealthDay, Washington Post, Los Angeles Times, San Francisco Chronicle, Atlanta Journal-Constitution, WebMD, and more than 300 other media outlets have run the story.

The environment we live in is obviously important to our health and our lives. This kind of focused research helps point the way to a set of decisions about the environment that can help create better health for the future for us all.

It was good work, and it has created a new level of energy on an important topic.

So this week, I am celebrating our Kaiser Permanente researchers who cared enough about environmental health to cross the globe to do the studies that came up with that result.

Well done, research team.

Be well.

George

* * *

Background Note: Our Research Extends from Obesity, to Cancer Prevention, to Death Rates Predicted by Literacy Levels

As I keep saying, I do love our research agenda. The next letter celebrates several research findings.

Our researchers have revealed, uncovered, and discerned significant findings in a number of research areas. This particular letter ends with an astounding piece of research. Our researchers found that the death rate for congestive heart failure patients actually tripled for patients who had low levels of medical literacy.

That very powerful initial finding about medical literacy and dying will trigger further research both inside KP and in other care settings. It's an amazing piece of work.

Each of the topics in this letter deserved their own letter — but when we have roughly a thousand research publications a year and I only have 52 weeks to write weekly letters, it makes sense to clump the research celebrations a bit.

Celebrating Research Linking Medical Literacy to Mortality – May 6, 2011

Dear KP Colleagues,

Kaiser Permanente researchers continue to hit home runs.

A recent study — published in the International Journal of Obesity — showed that people who got the right amount of sleep and had lower levels of stress were more likely to be successful in losing weight.

On the one hand, that doesn't seem like surprising information — but it was only speculation until Kaiser Permanente researchers did the study to prove that it was true.

More than 750 news outlets ran that story.

Another study using KP data found an association between the use of ACE inhibitors and an increased risk of breast cancer recurrence.

That piece of information was published online in the journal Breast Cancer Research and Treatment — and there were roughly 70 follow-up media pieces done on the topic.

Another KP study — one that was published in the Journal of Urology in March — showed an increased risk of erectile dysfunction in men who regularly take certain over-the-counter pain killers.

That research was covered in more than 160 media sites, including USA Today, Reuters, and the Los Angeles Times.

Each of those studies will add to the science of medicine.

One of the great advantages of our wonderful automated database is that we can search through large amounts of information to answer important medical questions. As an example, people wanted to know if Pioglitazone was associated with common cancers in people with diabetes. Very few care teams or medical researchers could answer that question. We could.

We reviewed two years of data for 252,467 patients to look for 10 key cancers. The result was published in the April issue of Diabetes Care. Our data showed no link... and our researchers then suggested that it would be a really good thing to do to look again for linkages at five and 10 years.

So for that study, we didn't find a link, and that was a good finding to have.

On another study, however, we found a clear link that pointed to a higher risk of death, and it was a link no one else had ever found.

That particular study was published this month. It will get fewer mass media reprints but it offers very useful information that may save lives. The study was done by our Colorado care team.

The new study very insightfully related medical literacy by individual patients to patient mortality rates. We learned that the death rate was higher for patients with low literacy scores. Our KP care team tested congestive heart failure (CHF) patients for their medical literacy level by asking each patient a couple of questions.

The patients then received a medical literacy score based on those questions.

The death rate was almost three times higher — 17.6 percent compared to 6.3 percent — for the people with the lowest medical literacy scores.

No one had ever identified that linkage before.

What does that piece of research tell us?

It tells us that we may have discovered a new and useful predictive tool to use that might help us help our CHF patients survive better and longer.

Saving lives is a very good thing to do. Determining that a specific patient might be at higher risk of dying is a very good thing to do.

That is definitely important and innovative research. It actually may open up whole new fields of research opportunity — linking medical literacy levels in patients to other health outcomes.

So my letter this week celebrates our total research teams. It also celebrates the folks who are trying to help CHF patients live longer by testing medical literacy levels to find out which patients are most at risk.

Again — well done.

Be well.

George

* * *

Background Note: Sometimes Our Research Teams are Needed to Show Whether Something in Care Delivery Really Works

Sometimes there are treatments in health care that are widely used across the entire country and even the world, but people who deliver care actually do not know for a fact whether those treatments work well or not at all. The Institute of Medicine is currently writing a couple of major reports for the country on science-based care. The IOM is developing strategies to deal with those issues and will be offering advice to everyone about how to have American health care evolve to becoming more of a "science-based" and "continuously learning" health care system. Both of those learning agendas exist now at KP, and they are described in my next letter.

One of the most lovely things about having a large database about the ongoing care of a lot of patients is that we can look at enough patient outcomes to figure out whether a given treatment is actually effective or whether it either damages patients or does no good at all. Answers to all of those questions are needed to make care better.

Our research into the effectiveness of the shingles vaccine was one of those efforts. That research is the topic of my next celebration letter.

Celebrating Our Shingles Vaccination Research – January 21, 2011

Dear KP Colleagues,

Shingles can really make a person miserable.

The pain and itching and the sheer levels of personal discomfort and deeply unpleasant skin irritation that can result from a case of shingles are something that many people absolutely hate and some people fear.

Shingles can ruin a week or a month and even a year; particularly when the case is severe and the symptoms refuse to go away.

Shingles is a form of herpes — herpes zoster — and in a bad case, it can be like having cold sores across expanses of the patient's body.

More than one million people a year get shingles in this country.

Why am I writing about shingles in my weekly letter?

We just made a major contribution to the body of science that relates to the treatment of herpes.

What did we do? We studied the actual impact of the new shingles vaccine on our patients.

We looked into our medical records and we studied 300,000 patients. We can do that level of study because our electronic medical record creates a magnificent database for medical research.

What did we learn?

We learned that the new shingles vaccine actually does work. But, not all of the time.

People did not know how well the vaccine worked. Initial studies had indicated that it worked at least some of the time. But our doctors also knew it absolutely did not work all of the time, because a number of people who have been given the vaccine still got shingles.

The vaccine obviously doesn't work perfectly. So the question we wanted and needed to answer was — how well did it work?

The answer is — it works well enough to reduce the number of shingles cases by 55 percent.

Fifty-five percent is a lot.

Shingles is such a pain that reducing the number of cases by more than half is a very good thing.

Baby boomers are particularly susceptible to shingles right now, because any immunity to the disease that happened early in life for baby boomers as the result of a case of childhood chicken pox tends to wear off by the golden years.

So 50 million baby boomers who are currently headed for a higher risk of shingles need to know what Kaiser Permanente researchers have just learned — you can reduce your shingles risk by more than half by using the vaccine.

The world outside Kaiser Permanente was hungry for that piece of information. More than 400 news media articles ran stories about our shingles research the first week after the study was published.

Jump to USA Today Article.

Major news media articles across the world covered the story. The USA Today article that is on this link was typical. Millions of people who might not have gotten that vaccination will probably now get it because that research was both done and well publicized.

Any time we can improve people's lives, it is a good thing. Improving lives for millions of people is a very good thing. The vaccine costs a couple of hundred dollars per dose. That's not cheap. But as the ad campaign says, the value of not getting a case of shingles is "priceless."

So my letter this week celebrates our researchers who took the time to do the study that showed the world that the vaccination works. We should also, I think, celebrate the fact that we have a patient care database that lets us do that kind of research.

Lives are better. Again.

Well done.

Be well.

George

✿ ✿ ✿

Background Note: Sometimes We Show That Suspected Links Do Not Exist

As I noted in the last letter, sometimes the most useful research we can do for the world involves research that either shows that a treatment does not work or research that shows a suspected linkage between two factors actually does not exist. Verifying real links is a valuable thing. Showing that suspected links do not exist can be equally valuable.

Because we have such a lovely database, we can do research in both directions. The next letter celebrates both links that we have found and links that we did not find.

The science of care delivery is improved by each of those findings. Data is a wonderful thing.

The autism links mentioned in the next letter were not even suspected until we did that research. Almost no one else has consistent and complete data about both children and new mothers. We have both sets of data for a lot of families, so we can learn some extremely important things that would never have been discovered if the research was done in settings that did not have both sets of data.

Celebrating KP Researchers Using our Data to Learn Whether Links Exist – April 6, 2012

Dear KP Colleagues,

Sometimes the most important thing that a medical research study shows is that there is some kind of link that is related to some specific factor that causes a disease or creates damage for patients.

That research can be golden. Showing that a specific chemical increases the risk of cancer, for example, is a valuable thing to learn. Finding links is important work.

But sometimes the most important finding of medical research is learning that a suspected link actually does not exist.

When people suspect that a link exists between some occurrence and a disease or a bad health outcome, there can be a tendency to be cautious and to avoid whatever is suspected of causing the bad outcome. In that case, medical science can add a lot of value by showing that the suspected link isn't a real link. Medical science and care delivery are both better when that research can be done.

Our researchers just disproved one of those suspected linkages. Quite a few caregivers had become concerned that the measles vaccine might be triggering febrile convulsions in children.

An earlier study had shown that one- to two-year-old kids actually did have higher levels of febrile convulsions that were related to measles vaccinations. Our researchers checked to see if the two issues were still linked in older kids... kids from four to six years old.

Our researchers took a look at our database to see if that same link also existed for the older kids.

A database is a lovely thing.

The beauty of a database is that it can contain facts about care that can help us understand important things about care that we can only guess at without actual data.

We have a lovely database at Kaiser Permanente, so we did take a look to see if older kids with those particular shots were having an undue number of convulsions.

What did we learn?

We learned a lot.

We now know that the measles vaccine does not create any difference in the rate of those seizures in children between the ages of 4 and 6 years.

We did that study, and we shared those results with the world. More than 100 media outlets — including US News and World Report, Medscape, and WebMD — ran the story.

Now other caregivers can have peace of mind about that risk for children in that age category.

Finding out that links do not exist is important work. We often do it well because we have great data.

We did earlier research that showed vaccines did not increase the risk of autism. We had access to significant amounts of data for that study. A lot of people had been deeply concerned about that issue of autism being associated with vaccinations, so that was also very good research to do.

Our data showed that link did not exist.

Our research data also provided reassurance about the safety of ADHD medications after concerns regarding their possible link to serious cardiovascular events.

Again — some people who had heart problems also had taken those medications. Other people in health care had suspicions. We had data. Our KP researchers found that, overall, those taking ADHD drugs were no more likely to have a heart attack, stroke or sudden death, compared with a matched group of non-users.

We had significant numbers of real patients. Many medical research studies that use paper medical records as their input data source can only look at two or three hundred patients. Paper files hide a lot of science and cripple opportunities for learning because paper records are so hard to use for research.

Our researchers compared two decades' worth of health records for 150,000 adults who were on one of these medications to the records of 300,000 adults who weren't on those medications, to arrive at their results.

Another KP de-linking study dealt with the concern that women who took ACE inhibitor drugs might be putting their children at risk of birth defects. People were very worried about that possible outcome.

What did we learn?

We looked at more than 465,000 births — a huge database — and we discovered that those drugs were not causing birth defects.

Likewise, our research on the impact of the whooping cough vaccine also showed that kids were not being damaged by that vaccination. We helped get rid of that fear, as well.

Sometimes we do find links. We did learn from our research that the age of parents — particularly the age of fathers — did increase the risk of autism. Fathers over 40 are 50 percent more likely to have autistic children. That was good to know.

Another important study showed that the risk of autism increased 200 percent when pregnant women took certain prescription drugs in the first trimester of their pregnancy. That was also good to know. Other researchers are now building on our insights in that area.

So sometimes, our studies do find solid links. Links do exist. But for the measles vaccine and our most current research, we were able to create peace of mind for the medical community that the suspected link with febrile seizures does not exist. That was a lovely contribution for our team to make to medical science.

So this week, I am celebrating the latest work of our KP researchers who dispelled the concern about that suspected link and made care better-informed as a result. It's good for the world to know that link does not exist.

Well done.

Be well.

George

☆ ☆ ☆

Background Note: DNA is the Next Research Frontier

The next major area of progress in medical science and medical research may well have genetic components. We believe strongly that DNA research is on the cusp of a golden age for care improvement.

DNA-based insights about patient risk levels will help us anticipate diseases for patients so we can prevent them. DNA research will also help us figure out the best treatments for many patients. We already know that a number of drugs work very well for people with a particular DNA set and that those same treatments can create a dangerous delay in getting to good care for other patients.

DNA science will make us a lot smarter, and we will be able to deliver better care when we know more about the genetic reality for specific patients and groups of patients. We strongly believe that to be true.

We also believe that we are particularly well suited to be a major scientific player in that new care improvement research era because of our electronic medical records. We have real patient data that can be linked to DNA data at a scope and scale that simply doesn't exist in almost any other setting.

So we intend to do some of that very important research — with full and clear approval and individual permission from our members and from the patients whose DNA is on file in our laboratories and storage units. Full disclosure and clear patient approval levels are the solid foundation for that work.

We have been blessed with a good number of members who have — with full disclosure and with full understanding — given us their DNA samples and agreed to give us permission to do that research. Those patients really want medical science to get better and lives to be saved. Those patients deserve our collective gratitude. We are all in their scientific debt.

I have included a couple of celebration letters about our efforts on DNA related research in this book. Those letters were also fun to write.

Celebrating the Addition of DNA Data to Our Medical Research Tool Kit – April 9, 2010

Dear KP Colleagues,

We just achieved an important and historic breakthrough in our efforts aimed at creating the world's best tool kit for medical research.

We have now collected DNA data for more than 130,000 of our members. In total, more than 400,000 Kaiser Permanente members have joined the research program allowing us to collect their DNA data for the good of medical science. We have begun the process of collecting DNA samples from those members and we have now actually collected data from 138,000 people. That is a lot of DNA.

Iceland now has one of the largest DNA datasets in the world with about 112,000 DNA samples — and the data from Iceland is from a population a lot less diverse than the Northern California population of Kaiser Permanente. Our DNA database is unique compared to most other databases in the world because it comes from such a diverse population and because we can link the DNA data to our electronic health records database to do important research.

Why are we doing this level of DNA research? To learn. And to improve care.

These are exciting times for medical research. We will be able to take our new dataset and learn wonderful new things. We now know, for example, from really good earlier Kaiser Permanente research that being significantly overweight and having very high cholesterol levels in our thirties and forties can increase our personal risk of dementia in our sixties and seventies by roughly 260 percent. We learned about that set of connections by combining our old historical medical files from decades ago with our new electronic KP HealthConnect® dataset for patients who are still with us after all these years to figure out that dementia risk and mid-life body fat have a major statistical association.

That's just the start. DNA will take us to another, higher level of learning. With our new DNA dataset and our almost unique ability to look at mid-life risk factors, we should eventually be able to figure out exactly which people are most at risk for dementia and Alzheimer's based on their mid-life cholesterol levels.

Odds are very good that we will be able to learn something very useful from that work. The number of Alzheimer's cases in America is exploding. We might be able to learn a lot more about why that is happening and — very importantly — we might be able to tell our own individual patients — "you are genetically at a very high risk of Alzheimer's and you can cut your personal risk by more than half by keeping your cholesterol levels low."

I have mentioned that possibility to audiences and have asked people if they would like to know if their own DNA made them 3.6 times more likely to have dementia if they had high cholesterol and a larger abdomen. Just about everyone in each audience says they would definitely like to know that information about their personal risk levels.

The DNA data will let us do some important learning.

We did an important analysis from our old database a couple of years ago that told us patients who were taking Vioxx were quite a bit more likely to die of heart attacks. We took Vioxx off our formulary and we told the world what we had learned and what we had done.

Other data reinforced our findings and Vioxx was pulled entirely off the market.

That example is often cited as one of the evidences for the value that our dataset creates.

My own suspicion is that our new DNA dataset will allow us to take that risk analysis another important step forward to see if Vioxx is very dangerous for some people and not dangerous at all for other people.

Vioxx might be a great and entirely safe drug for some people — but we don't know which ones because our old dataset only had macro numbers about the increased number of deaths and could not — and did not — tell us who, genetically, was most likely to die.

It may be that the drug had the same impact on everyone. It also might be that some people would benefit with no risk and some other people would be at major risk.

That would be good to know.

This is incredibly exciting work. We are pointed in exactly the right direction. Our researchers will be the envy of the medical research world because we will be able to ask and answer questions that other researchers can only wish they could either ask or answer.

So my letter this week celebrates the Northern California team of researchers who are putting together our new DNA data library — and the teams of researchers all across Kaiser Permanente who will be able to take that data to do some of the most important research in the history of health care.

Be well.

George

* * *

Celebrating 170,000 DNA Samples in Our New Biorepository – September 9, 2011

Dear KP Colleagues,

Medical research for the entire world, for a very long time, has almost always been done on a very limited scale — with a very narrow focus for almost every research project.

Medical research has been extremely slow. Years of focused study are often needed to figure out a very narrow range of findings about just a single and narrow medical topic.

Most studies have also involved only a few hundred people — and most studies done in most settings have been rigidly time limited — with the learning and data gathering ending and then truncated for each study immediately after the funded research expires. Research tends to be very expensive, and funding sources tend to limit funds available for any given project.

Given all of those challenges and constraints, it's a miracle that medical research happens at all — and it's a further miracle that very much is learned when those old-school, traditionally structured research projects do happen.

Those constraints define the bad old days of research.

To make matters even more challenging for the bad old days, almost all medical research has been done in the context of paper medical records — with a separate paper record folder for each doctor for each patient. Paper records mean that the basic data collected about each patient tends to be limited, isolated, utterly inert, and generally hard to access.

Some of the most exciting potential opportunities for medical research relate to genetics and the DNA impact for both disease and the risk of disease. The potential learning in those areas of medical science are huge, but data on the relationships of genetic factors to any given set of medical issues, risks, or opportunities has been almost impossible to obtain — and basic DNA research has been extremely expensive — because it has been just plain too hard to have credible data in significant volume about a sufficient number of patients.

To be useful for research on health, DNA samples and genetic data have to be linkable to high quality, comprehensive data on disease and treatment of disease. That level of linked data is still extremely rare and difficult for many researchers to access.

It has been very difficult for researchers to relate DNA data to the care issues and the care needs of any statistically credible sample of patients.

Medical science and the application of DNA learning to medical science have been severely handicapped by all of these logistical and financial factors.

That's the bad news.

The good news is that we are now on the cusp of a golden age for medical research for medical care in the world.

The very good news is that the cutting edge for a new golden age of research is probably us — Kaiser Permanente.

We have the potential at Kaiser Permanente to completely transform research. We have a wonderful team of world-class medical researchers. Our researchers have the medical information for all of our patients on the computer — not just in paper files.

We have electronic access to large amounts of data, and we have also kept longitudinal records of patient care over time, because we are a care system, and we have maintained these records to support care delivery.

We are now using that data to do some great research.

Our research teams have been able to figure out, for example, that the risk of Alzheimer's in your 60s goes up by more than 200 percent when you have high cholesterol and are overweight in your 40s.

No one even suspected that until we did the research. It took longitudinal data to figure that out.

We also now know that when mothers have an amniotic fluid infection during pregnancy, their children are much more likely to have asthma later in life. Again, no one even suspected that to be true until we did the research.

Anyone else trying to do that kind of research who did not have access to patient data in volume from an electronic medical record would not be able to do that level of research that linked the mothers to the children, and then related and linked diseases in the mothers to entirely different diseases in the children, and actually did that work with statistically credible research sample sizes.

We owe it to the world to do that level of research, because we are almost unique in being able to do that research, and that research needs to be done.

We owe it to the world to answer a whole range of questions that really need to be answered for medical science by medical research.

We don't have either a perfect data set or perfect access to data. That isn't yet possible. But we have extremely good data, and we now have very workable access to that data — so we are in the process of having a great, adventurous, exciting, and increasingly fruitful journey into whole new fields of medical research.

It's an exciting journey — and we want to continue down those paths of learning to the point where we can answer extremely important questions — questions like: "Why is the rate of autism growing so rapidly in this country and the world?"

We are already working on that exact issue.

Our autism studies have already added real value to modern science. We now know that when the mother-to-be takes certain drugs early in a pregnancy, that drug intake tends to increase the risk of kids being autistic. We also know from our research that older parents are more likely to have autistic kids.

The link to older mothers was discovered by other people, but our study was the first to find that both maternal and paternal age are independently associated with autism risk, and that the risk is somewhat higher for older dads than for older moms.

Data can have almost magical learning value.

So what exactly am I celebrating this week in my weekly letter?

DNA.

We are adding DNA to our Kaiser Permanente research tool kit. We are linking DNA to real data about care.

We have patients in our care system who have volunteered to help us create what might already be the largest nongovernmental DNA sample collection and database in the world.

We are collecting DNA samples every single day. We just hit a milestone in that collection journey.

We now have 170,000 individual DNA samples filed and archived in our new Northern California DNA repository.

We have conducted genome-wide genotyping on more than 100,000 of those DNA samples, testing over 675,000 single nucleotide polymorphisms on each sample of DNA.

We will now be doing research that will link genetic data from our members with data from their electronic medical records and also with an array of environmental and behavioral data.

Our goal is to do research to help us figure out how to deliver better care and how to improve public health by preventing or reducing the severity of disease.

The size and diverse composition of our 100,000 person sample and the high quality comprehensive data that are linked together make this an unprecedented resource for studies of genetic and environmental impacts on health and disease.

There is nothing like this anywhere in the world. It makes it possible to simultaneously conduct research on many different diseases and health conditions, and to investigate effects on response to medications.

The National Institutes of Health has been a major source of funding for our efforts to genotype 100,000 members. Foundations such as the Robert Wood Johnson Foundation, the Ellison Medical Foundation, and the Wayne and Gladys Valley Foundation have provided generous support for building the research program and collecting DNA samples.

We are receiving all that support from those important organizations because people in national health care research circles appreciate how valuable the combined KP database and KP delivery of care is to the learning process for health care. We have received millions of dollars in funding to gather the samples, genotype them, and create a research resource that links the resulting data to electronic medical records of patients who have volunteered to be part of this research.

We are at the very beginning of that learning curve. It's an exciting place to be. The outside world agrees that it is an exciting effort. More than 100 media outlets wrote stories about our new DNA database when we achieved the milestone of 100,000 samples. Here is one of those stories.

So my letter this week celebrates that special Kaiser Permanente milestone event — achieving and exceeding 170,000 DNA samples, and actually genotyping for over 100,000 samples. All that data is now set up as a deposit and resource for future medical science learning and discovery.

We don't even know what we don't know about DNA and health right now. But we are on a path to learn. So my letter this week celebrates all of the people who are doing the work to take us down the road to the next multiple generations of medical learning — and who have put in place a database biorepository of 170,000 DNA samples that is a resource for the world.

Be well.

George

✿ ✿ ✿

Background Note: Medicare Decided to Rate All Health Plans Using 53 Measures of Quality, Access, and Service

An increasing number of outside organizations now rate and evaluate our performance as a health care organization, as a provider of care, and as a health plan.

We tend to do really well in those outside evaluations.

The next letter, for example, celebrates KP's performance on the Medicare 5-star rating system. Medicare set up what might be the toughest set of measurement criteria for any major buyer of health care on the planet. Medicare decided to use 53 separate, clearly defined criteria to compare quality levels and service levels at all Medicare health plans.

They rated 459 Medicare Advantage plans across the country. They gave the top plans in the country five stars, and the lowest plans one star. The scorecard isn't easy. Only nine health plans in the entire country earned the full 5 stars.

How well did we do? We did really well.

We earned five full stars for 90 percent of our Medicare members.

Our lowest score was 4.5 stars. Our larger regions all earned the full five stars. We had the most 5-star health plans in the country by a wide margin.

The next letter celebrates our 5-star success level. When Medicare looks at all of those criteria and selects the top plans in the country for quality and service, it's a really good thing to be at the top of that list.

Celebrating Our Highest Quality Medicare Star Ratings for Quality and Service – October 14, 2011

Dear KP Colleagues,

Stars make a difference.

Stars matter for Medicare.

Medicare now rates all Medicare Advantage plans in the country with a one- to five-star rating. They announced their star ratings for the year earlier this week.

Five stars is the best.

Only nine health plans in the entire country received five-star ratings.

How did we do?

Five of our regions earned five stars.

Our three regions who did not receive five-star ratings earned 4.5 stars.

Four-point-five stars is also a great score on a five-star rating.

The other five-star plans in the country also, not surprisingly, tend to be health plans with close provider/plan linkages. Group Health Co-op in Seattle is an affiliate of ours. They earned five stars, as well.

Other winning plans were in Massachusetts, Maine, and Wisconsin. We are the only five-star plans in our regions.

What will happen as a result of the five-star rating? Several things — all good. The government will tell seniors who want to enroll in a Medicare Advantage plan how many stars each plan has.

The rating system will be very visible to people who want to enroll in Medicare Advantage plans. We will also be a bit more visible to everyone who works in health care quality and service agendas in America because the five-star plan is unique in the country as a measure of both care and quality. And people in the quality world know what it means to earn five stars.

It's a tough scoring system. Medicare measures plans for about 50 different performance categories. The performance categories include helping patients stay healthy, managing chronic conditions, and objectively measured member satisfaction. Service level scores are extremely important.

Public recognition is not the only advantage that comes from earning five stars. Enrollment rules change, as well, for five-star plans.

Up until now, Medicare Advantage plans have only had one seven-week enrollment period each year when new members can choose to join plans.

That relatively short open enrollment period is when the big enrollment push for all Medicare Advantage plans happens.

At KP, we gear up. We run ads, set up telephone sales teams, send out mailings, and work hard to take advantage of that Medicare Advantage enrollment window before it closes. When the window is over, enrollment ends, except for people who turn 65 and become newly Medicare eligible.

Now — for the first time ever — Medicare has decided not to close that enrollment window for any plan that earns five stars.

Our five-star plans can now enroll new Medicare members all year.

All year is good.

Our Medicare programs are important to us. We have over a million total members from Medicare. We obviously deliver star-quality service and care to those members.

The Medicare Advantage program is a really good fit for Kaiser Permanente because seniors often have multiple health conditions and need team care, and team care is a special competency of Kaiser Permanente.

So this is all very good news.

The world can look at our new star ratings and see how objective outside people and quantifiable scoring systems rate our care processes, our operations, and our service.

Our successes in those areas will be visible to the world and extremely relevant to our future.

So this week, with great pleasure, I am celebrating stars. The California, Northwest, Hawaii, and Colorado regions earned five stars. The Georgia, Ohio, and Mid-Atlantic States regions earned 4.5 stars.

Only a very tiny number of other plans in the entire country earned as many stars as Kaiser Permanente. As the CEO of one of those five-star plans said to me in an e-mail yesterday — "We had stars — you guys have a constellation."

Well done, Kaiser Permanente. It took all of our caregivers and all of our plan teams and all of our support staff working together to make these star-rating successes happen.

Five stars.

Well done.

Be well.

George

* * *

Background Note: J.D. Power and Associates Also Gave us No. 1 Ratings

As I noted before, Medicare rated us highly. Five stars is a great score.

We also were rated highly by J.D. Power and Associates — the organization that evaluates customer satisfaction and product quality. J.D. Power rated us in three areas. They rated us in customer satisfaction as a health plan for employer groups, for individual members, and they rated us in customer satisfaction as a mail-order pharmacy system.

How did we do?

In 2011, we were rated number one in all categories. We were rated number one again as a health plan in our service areas, and we were rated number one again for our pharmacy mail-order system.

Number one is the right number.

The first of two following letters celebrates one of our 2011 J.D. Power and Associates wins for customer satisfaction.

The letter that follows is the 2009 Celebration Letter that discusses our top rated mail-order pharmacy program — that was the first year of our three consecutive yearly wins in that category.

For this year — 2012 — J.D. Power released their ratings for the accolade ranking us number one in employer group customer satisfaction as a health plan for all of our larger regions. And our 2012 scores with employers were even better than they were when I wrote the following 2011 letter.

We also did well in the individual member satisfaction rating. J.D. Power ranked us highest in that category in March, as well, for all of our larger regions.

So the things we are doing to make care better and to support the buyers who chose us as their health plan seems to be working well.

Celebrating Our J.D. Power Win and Zero Injuries – July 1, 2011

Dear KP Colleagues,

A week ago, I mentioned that my favorite number was one. I love it when we are number one.

A couple of folks suggested that my favorite number should be zero — like having zero serious pressure ulcers at one of our hospitals, or zero central line infections.

Zero is a great number, too. In some ways, zero is better than one — because one is comparative and zero is absolute.

Zero isn't relative. Zero means we are doing something so well that we can't get a better score than that.

One means we beat everyone else who is being scored. We could have dozens of broken bones and still have the lowest numbers and still be the best and be rated as number one. In that case, one is very good, and it isn't zero.

So what is my favorite number? I have decided to use the same standard for favorite number that I use for favorite son... recognizing that I can have more than one favorite.

And just to show for a fact that I love both numbers equally, I am celebrating one of each this week.

Let's start with the number one.

J.D. Power and Associates is a research company. They survey the marketplace on a lot of issues and performances levels. They look at how the marketplace responds to various products and companies. People respect the solid work that J.D. Power does.

They just surveyed more than 7,000 businesses who buy health coverage — employers — and asked those 7,000 employers to rate their satisfaction with their health plans.

How did we do?

Since this letter is celebrating both one and zero — and since zero on that service survey is not a possible score — I suspect you know how we were rated on employer satisfaction among health plans.

We were rated Number One.

We beat the number two plan by 27 points on a 1,000 point rating scale.

Employers who buy our coverage rate us number one in the region for satisfaction based on service to their employees, service to the employer, and meeting their needs.

This service level is really important to us, because those employers have a lot of choices of health plans. Other plans want to steal our members and turn our patients into their patients. If we were to underperform on service, we could see other health coverage competitors winning more often, because employers decide every year who their health plan options will be.

So having those employers rate us as number one is a solid win for us. I suspect we will celebrate and share that rating with the consultants who give advice to employers — and we will share it with the employers themselves — thanking them both for giving us access to their employees as patients and for continuing to offer our coverage.

That's my number one celebration this week — best in service for employers.

What is the zero?

We just had an excellent zero at our Baldwin Park hospital.

We are a health care organization. We take care of people. Our goal is to heal people, repair people, and keep people healthy.

We really do not want to ever damage people — and we very much do not want to have our own staff damaged by being injured on the job.

Workplace injuries are not a good thing. People in health care do get injured. We have lifting injuries, muscle strains, falls, cuts, needle sticks, and a number of other mishaps and damages that can happen on the job.

We are learning to get better at preventing injuries and at not having those kinds of workplace injuries happen. Causing those injuries to be massively reduced involves the same kind of consistent best practices and commitment that gets our pressure ulcers down to zero in our highest performing care sites.

We have lift teams, focused safety agendas, and we have high-performing unit-based teams focusing on workplace safety across KP.

So how are we doing?

We are getting better. We are learning, paying attention, helping each other, and getting better every month.

We now have a best site that has achieved a zero.

I love zero.

Our Baldwin Park Hospital went the entire month of March this year without one single workplace injury that was at the level defined by the workplace injury process as an injury.

Zero.

Zero is a great number.

Zero injuries can be done.

Good people worked hard to prevent injuries on that site, and that effort succeeded.

Well done.

So my letter this week celebrates both being rated number one on service in a survey of more than 7,000 employers across the nation and having a care site so focused on workplace injuries that we have achieved zero injuries for a complete and entire month.

It's a lot like my own kids — I do have more than one favorite.

Be well.

George

✳ ✳ ✳

Celebrating Our Pharmacy Teams – September 25, 2009

Dear KP Colleagues,

A few years ago, we decided to make getting prescriptions refilled easier for a lot of our members and patients by setting up a mail-based distribution service.

We were one of the first organizations to pioneer mail refills for prescriptions. We experimented, learned, changed, expanded, and enhanced our processes with our members' needs and convenience foremost in our mind.

Today, quite a few organizations have followed our lead and distribute prescriptions by mail.

In fact, there are so many organizations doing that work that there is actually a national study that compares how all of those systems do.

I suspect that you suspect where this letter is going. We have just been ranked. J.D. Power and Associates does the ranking. They actually rank pharmacy programs in four categories — chain stores, mass merchandisers, supermarkets, and mail-order pharmacies. We compete in the mail-order pharmacy category.

So how did we do?

We won in our segment.

Out of a possible 1,000 points, we scored 877. That was the highest score for mail-order competitors.

It was also the highest score in any category. Health Mart won the chain store category with 864 points. Target won mass merchandisers with 831 points. Wegmans won the supermarket category with 865 points. So our 877 was a pretty good score.

Members love mail-order pharmacy for the sheer convenience of not having to drive to some geographic location to pick up their medications.

It just makes sense. It saves time and travel — and we have focused well enough on making that process functionally better that we have climbed the ladder to first place — against some tough and well-known competitors. In the first half of 2009, we have already filled 3.2 million prescriptions by mail. That's a lot of member trips to the pharmacy that didn't have to happen.

So that's my celebration this week. The fact that we met our members' needs and expectations in prescription pharmacy so well that our members rated us number one. Nice when that happens.

Be well.

George

✿ ✿ ✿

Background Note: We also did Well on the National Brand Credibility Rating

We had the best performance scores with Medicare in their 5-star competition, and we also had number-one scores with J.D. Power and Associates on customer satisfaction levels as a health plan in five regions. Consumer Reports scores can be looked up by anyone on the Internet.

So we have had some major wins in performance, service, satisfaction, and quality.

One question that is created by all of the performance wins is — how are we doing relative to our credibility as a brand? If we win on our actual performance, how are we regarded as a credible organization by consumers and members?

The good news is that we are also seeing some very nice positioning relative to our brand credibility.

A well-regarded measurement organization called Satmetrix actually measures brand credibility and customer satisfaction for major companies across multiple industries.

The Satmetrix people recently rated us number one in our industry. That number-one brand credibility rating also was worth a celebration letter to the people of Kaiser Permanente.

Celebrating KP Top Ranking in Consumer Loyalty and Value – March 30, 2012

Dear KP Colleagues,

What do Apple, Vanguard, Trader Joe's, Amazon.com, and Virgin America have in common with Kaiser Permanente?

Those are the organizations that were each just rated number one in the country in their industries for consumer loyalty and overall value by their customers.

The evaluation was done by Satmetrix, using a survey of more than 30,000 people who all said they had significant experience with a company or product.

We won overwhelmingly for health care plans. We were rated number one. The average score for all health plans in the survey was four.

Our score was 33.

We beat our closest health plan competitor by 16 points.

What does that tell us?

Last week, I wrote a letter about the 15 wonderful Kaiser Permanente quality of care programs that were nominated for this year's James A. Vohs Award for Quality.

Each of those programs is a wonderful way of improving care. Those were just the 2012 nominees.

We have a whole array of programs at Kaiser Permanente that save many lives and advance both the science of care and the practice of care every single day.

I suspect that the health plan competitors who finished behind us on the Satmetrix scores have almost nothing that compares with those 15 quality programs.

Our members know that we really do care deeply about getting care right.

Our sepsis death prevention programs may be the best in the world.

Our pressure ulcer avoidance programs also are world class. Our safety programs are getting continuously better and we will keep getting better.

We are working hard to make the right thing easy to do in multiple areas — including care connectivity.

Our new smartphone app had one million users in the first month after its release.

We are now doing a million e-visits between our doctors and our patients every month.

We have over 20 HEDIS scores where the top health plan in the country for quality is Kaiser Permanente.

J.D. Power and Associates also just ranked us highest in member satisfaction among health plans in all five of our larger regions.

J.D. Power and Associates has also ranked our mail-order pharmacy highest in customer satisfaction in the country.

We are doing a lot of things right.

We are saving lives, and we are focusing on our patients in powerful and effective ways.

We know we are working hard to do the right things.

So it is good when an outside organization that evaluates how well organizations are regarded by their customers discovers that our members rate us more highly than other health plans that are rated by their members.

Apple and Amazon and Trader Joe's are good company to be in.

Number one is the right ranking.

So my letter this week celebrates all of the people at Kaiser Permanente who let each of our members and each of our patients know every day that we care and that we are doing the right things for the right reasons and doing them well.

Satmetrix is a good win to have.

Well done.

Be well.

George

* * *

Background Note: When We Need Our Computers to Perpetually Perform, Then Uptime and Shadow Read Are both Wonderful Wins

We rely heavily on our computers to support the delivery of care. There may be very few care systems on the planet who get more use out of their computer-based tool kit. We are winning awards with the results of our computer supported team care. Our computers are at the heart of much of what we do.

So we obviously need our computers to be available — all of the time. We take that availability need very seriously. We have committed to making availability be a core competency of ours as an organization.

We clearly need our computers to be functioning. We place a high value on our computer support tools for care and we need those tools to be available to our caregivers when patients need care.

So we assign a very high operational and functional priority at Kaiser Permanente on systems availability. We work very hard to keep our computer centers functioning at all times, and we work very hard to maintain high levels of systems access and availability.

So how well are we doing in those efforts?

We are doing well.

We actually have earned a couple of additional awards in those areas. The Uptime Institute looks at computer processes in all industries and gives recognition to the computer sites that are up all the time. Banks and financial institutes tend to win those Uptime awards. No other health care provider has won any Uptime awards.

We have now won seven.

The attached celebration letter recognized our uptime achievements. This is an old letter — recognizing our very first uptime win. I have written other letters since that time to celebrate our continued uptime wins — because we keep winning them.

I included that particular letter in this book because it also celebrates our unique "Shadow Read" capability that keeps the data on patients available in the local care sites if the linkages to the central computer facility are down. "Shadow Read" was a brilliant piece of work that, in retrospect, I should have celebrated with a separate letter.

Celebrating Our Continuous Availability – January 29, 2010

Dear KP Colleagues,

When patient care is supported by computers, it's important that the computers be available.

"Down time" is bad when the computers that are down are the computers that doctors and other caregivers need to help deliver care.

The perfect system for care should have all of the information about all of the patients, and the data should be available all of the time.

The goal of computer-supported care should be real-time care data.

So we are working toward that goal at Kaiser Permanente with our KP HealthConnect® system. We probably have more patient data on the computer than anyone in health care.

We also lead the world in computer connectivity with our patients. More than 160,000 of our members connect to our caregivers and to our computer systems each and every single day.

So our goal is a functioning computer system that is available 24 hours a day, 365 days a year, with zero downtime.

So how are we doing? That is what I am celebrating this week.

The Uptime Institute — a national organization that reviews computer systems' availability — just announced its 2009 winners for their Continuous Availability Awards.

The awards are given to data centers.

To be considered for the Continuous Availability Award, companies must have a minimum of one full year of 100 percent data center infrastructure continuous availability to their customers — and they must clearly state their commitment to availability to their customers.

Not 99.9 percent for the data center — 100 percent continuous data center availability.

So how did we do?

For 2009, only 16 member companies in the entire country received Continuous Availability Awards.

Of the 16 companies that received the award, only one was a health care organization. That one was us.

And we won the award for a couple of our data centers... two of our data centers where we run our electronic medical record and our patient connectivity systems.

Our Napa data center received a one-year award. Our Corona data center received two consecutive awards — because that data center was continuously available for the last two years.

That is round-the-clock support for our members.

These awards are given for the entire data center being continuously available. We also measure how well we do in keeping each piece of the data center available.

Our success rate in availability for our KP HealthConnect system for 2009 exceeded 99.9 percent. We had a few times when pieces of the KP HealthConnect system were temporarily down in some care sites — but our "Shadow Read" backup system filled in to keep the needed data available to our care teams for on-site patient care.

"Shadow Read" is actually a great program that deserves its own celebration.

Being available whenever our members need us is a top priority for us as a caregiving organization.

So my letter this week celebrates the teams that work tirelessly to keep our system sites and our care systems constantly available.

Winning three "Continuous Availability" awards, when no one else in health care delivery has ever won the award, shows other care sites that it is possible. That, all by itself, is a contribution because we are showing other health care organizations what can be done.

Absolute perfection does not happen. But we can come close. And all of us — caregivers and patients — deeply value system reliability, dependability, and availability.

Well done, IT team.

Be well.

George

* * *

Background Note: Winning IT Awards is a Good Thing

Information Week just ranked us in the top 50 companies in the world relative to IT performance. Their rating included all companies from all industries — including all of the pure IT companies who do nothing but IT.

We prefer being number one in any ranking, but being in the top 50 is good enough for now across all of the IT companies in the world.

This next letter celebrates a number of our external IT recognitions. As earlier letters pointed out, our IT performance has been high enough that HIMSS (Healthcare Information and Management Systems Society) has recognized us at multiple levels for our performance. We have some number one rakings from HIMSS.

We have also been recognized by the Uptime Institute, by Computerworld, by Information Week, by Fast Company, and by CIO Magazine as a top IT shop.

We need our computer tools to do well. Great care is supported by great tools. It's a good thing when our IT performance and our IT total tool kit is good enough to be recognized externally at multiple levels.

I thought mentioning multiple recognitions related to our IT performance was worth a weekly letter of its own.

Celebrating Receiving the Davies Award for Overall IT Excellence – September 23, 2011

Dear KP Colleagues,

We continue to win awards for health care IT performance and innovation.

Last week, the Healthcare Information and Management Systems Society (HIMSS) — the largest health care IT association in the world — gave us their top award for health care IT excellence — the Davies Award.

We have been a major winner of other HIMSS awards over the past several years. Our hospitals have received some very special recognition. As you may remember from an earlier celebration letter, HIMSS rates and ranks about 2,000 hospitals across the country every year for each hospital's health care IT competence and completeness.

Their top award for hospital IT achievement is to be a Stage 7 hospital. As of last year, there were 60 Stage 7 hospitals in the world.

Thirty-five of the Stage 7 winners were us — Kaiser Permanente hospitals.

No KP hospital is lower than Stage 6. I am optimistic that we can get everyone to Stage 7 by next year.

The Davies Award wasn't awarded just for our hospital computer success.

The Davies Award was given to us for our overall IT excellence across all aspects of care delivery. They looked at our total use of IT across our entire spectrum of care.

It's a good award — and clearly visible recognition in the health care world. HIMSS has an annual meeting with over 20,000 attendees. The next meeting will be held in Feb. 2012. It's the largest health care IT conference in the world.

They will officially give us the Davies Award at that meeting.

HIMSS isn't the only outside organization recognizing our IT skill set.

We also now have won six awards from the Uptime Institute. That award is given for 100 percent availability of online performance of our actual data centers.

All major companies in the United States are eligible for that Uptime Institute award.

Fewer than 20 companies a year across all industries win that award. We are the only health care organization to ever win that award from the Uptime Institute — and we have won it six times for three separate computer sites.

Why is winning the Uptime Institute award important to us?

When we set up a health care infrastructure that is so fully and continuously supported by computers that our hospitals are granted Stage 7 recognition, it's really important to have IT systems available so that our care teams can have our patients' data on-screen — in the exam room or the emergency room — when that data is needed for their care.

We have built a significant computer resource at KP. Lives are saved because of that total care.

Having our entire array of system resources available to us also gives us a great opportunity to be innovative. We created our own internal innovation fund for technology back in 2008. We asked people inside KP with really good ideas to bring those ideas forward as innovation proposals.

More than 480 innovation proposals have been submitted. There are some really great ideas. As of last week, 59 of those ideas have been funded and a number have been operationalized — including ideas like our automated glycemic calculator that helps us care for hospital patients better and more efficiently than we could with a manual calculation. We also built a real-time data grid that predicts hospital capacity so that when we schedule procedures, we can decrease our patients' wait times. We also have set up — based on an innovation center proposal — SMS messaging for appointment reminders.

Our people have great ideas.

Some health care organizations that set up extensive IT support infrastructures find their bureaucracy-based programs can become rigid, inflexible, and even dictatorial in their internal use of their systems.

We, of course, are absolutely rigid on issues like patient privacy and data security. But when it comes to actually using the systems to serve and save our patients and to deliver better care, we want to encourage creativity and continuously improving levels of innovation.

We have very smart and innovative people at KP. The public needs us to be a resource in remaking pieces of care.

That level of KP internal innovation has also been given some external recognition in the IT world.

InformationWeek magazine has given us a couple of innovation awards — recognizing both our telemedicine and teleconsulting projects, for example, as being among the "Top 20 Innovative Ideas to Steal."

InformationWeek just ranked 500 companies all across the planet, and across all industries, for using innovative IT to make a notable difference in the way they do business.

How did we do on that international IT innovation scale?

We did well. Last week, they ranked us 34 out of the top 500 companies ranked across all industries across the globe.

Other parties have noticed our systems capabilities as well.

The research we are doing with our IT database has been recognized by organizations like the National Institutes of Health, and people at NIH know that we can do research that no one else in the health care world can do. We are expanding the use of our research with our new DNA registry.

We are doing lots of good stuff. People are noticing.

We also were ranked in CIO Magazine's CIO 100 list for our innovative use of information technology in our mobile care vans — and Fast Company magazine rated us the fifth most innovative health care company in the world.

In many ways, this is a good time to be us.

So winning the Davies Award last week was another nice recognition that we are doing some things right, and other people are noticing.

But more important than the award itself, the really important fact is that people and patients are benefitting from our IT tools every single day.

We are here to serve patients and to save lives. Our IT capabilities enhance our abilities to achieve these goals.

So my letter this week congratulates all of the folks who use our IT tools to provide great patient care — and all of the folks who foster and support and nurture and encourage our health care IT innovation — and also achieve our basic health care IT blocking and tackling.

Well done.

Be well.

George

✿ ✿ ✿

Background Note: Some State Governments Also Now Have Recognition Programs

State governments in a couple of our states also have begun rating and ranking health plans for their performance.

How are we doing? We have been rated in two states. We won both of them.

We have earned the highest scores for health plans for both California and Washington State.

Our performance scores keep getting better.

The next letter celebrates one of those state rating wins.

Celebrating Our Focus on Quality, Service and Preventing Obesity – February 12, 2010

Dear KP Colleagues,

There were a couple of interesting sets of news articles about us this week. The first set of articles were based on an annual scoring process for health plans created by the state of California.

The state rated all health plans in the state on both service and quality levels, and awarded one to four stars in multiple categories of performance to each plan.

We did well.

Our Southern California Region was the first health plan in the nine-year history of the scoring process to receive four stars for both quality and service.

Our Northern California Region had the highest scores in Northern California.

As the Sacramento Journal said on Tuesday, "Kaiser Permanente Northern California Region earned the highest rating for care standards, and three stars for member satisfaction. The HMO giant's Southern California operation collected four-star ratings in both categories, the only of the nine HMOs to earn the honor. Both Kaiser north and south had high marks for asthma and lung care, checking for cancer, Chlamydia screenings and diabetes, heart, maternity and mental health care."

The Orange County Journal naturally had a more "southern" perspective on the scores and wrote, "Kaiser Permanente in Southern California has received the highest ranking based on national standards of quality care and patient satisfaction, according to data released Tuesday by the California Office of the Patient Advocate.

The state compared data from patient medical records to national quality standards for the treatment of asthma, heart care and proper use of antibiotics. On the consumer side, the state looked at customer service, complaints and satisfaction with doctors."

More than forty other California news media outlets ran similar stories.

Those are good scores.

We are working hard to make sure that we are the best and the safest place for people to go for care. We have dozens of internal initiatives to improve care, improve patient safety, and improve service — and we are not yet at the levels we intend to achieve. But we are now the best in the world in a few areas, the best in the U.S. in some areas, and the best in each region in quite a few other areas.

And we have areas where we need to get better — for both care and service. We are very much focused on continuous improvement because people trust us with their lives and people trust us with their health — and that is a sacred sort of trust. We owe our patients and our members our best efforts — and we are moving nicely in those directions.

The latest California scorecard is a good external indicator that progress is being made.

We also had another very interesting and positive media exposure this week. The second set of articles ran in media outlets across the country.

In the middle of the snow storms and the terrible weather in Washington, D.C., First Lady Michelle Obama held a White House press conference Tuesday to announce a brand new, extremely important initiative to fight childhood obesity in America.

Childhood obesity is running at epidemic levels, and the lifetime consequences of that obesity are far too often damaging and sometimes cause horrible future health status and problems for each obese child.

So childhood obesity is a very serious and high priority issue for the country.

The First Lady had six co-sponsors for her initiative. Kaiser Permanente was one of the six partner organizations — selected because of our work in healthy eating, Thriving, and helping children deal with and avoid obesity.

We were recognized for our work in the White House. The President and First Lady also announced that a new independent foundation called "Partnership for a Healthier America" is being created by Kaiser Permanente, The California Endowment, Nemours, Robert Wood Johnson Foundation, WK Kellogg Foundation, and Alliance for a Healthier Generation, to guide and support the childhood obesity campaign.

We are in very good company. It is a great cause. America needs a future of better health, our children need better health, and we owe America our assistance in making that happen.

Think Thrive.

Congratulations to the KP teams who are making that whole health improvement agenda very real.

Be well.

George

✵ ✵ ✵

Background Note: Hospital Recognitions Continue to Grow

We are one of the largest hospital systems in this country, and — if you exclude the countries where the government owns all of the hospitals — we are actually one of the largest hospital systems in the world.

Our goal isn't to be the largest hospital system. Our goal is to be the best hospital system. We already have what might be the lowest death rates from the number-one cause of hospital death — sepsis. We rate among the lowest hospitals in the world relative to pressure ulcers, and we are doing great work on central-line infection prevention.

We are focused on safety and performance.

We are also as earlier letters pointed out, a winner in internal electronic connectivity inside our hospitals.

Our hospitals have received multiple recognitions. In addition to every Kaiser Permanente hospital receiving the highest rating from the Joint Commission (JCHO) rating process, and in addition to having a number of hospitals included in the Newsweek ratings of best hospitals, we have been recognized by the Leapfrog Group for our high levels of hospital performance.

The Leapfrog Group is a prestigious set of major American companies who want health care to "leapfrog" into a future of care excellence. They rate hospitals as part of their efforts to encourage and recognize best care.

My weekly letter celebrating our initial Leapfrog Group recognition follows. I expect to be able to write an even better letter about that recognition after their results next year are available.

Celebrating Our Hospital Care Teams – December 9, 2011

Dear KP Colleagues,

One of the most highly regarded hospital recognitions in America is the one done every year by the Leapfrog Group.

The Leapfrog Group is a national organization made up primarily of major employers who want American health care to "leapfrog" into a higher-quality future.

The Group is highly respected in American business and in national policy circles. They encourage care improvement at multiple levels.

One of their primary initiatives is an annual rating and ranking they do of American hospitals.

They rate quality, surgical outcomes, internal support systems, and they have set up stringent performance standards for a number of complex hospital procedures and processes.

There are more than 5,700 registered and licensed hospitals in America. The Leapfrog Group reviews nearly 1,200 of those hospitals — looking at the best performers. We were included in that review in the urban hospital category.

Slightly fewer than four percent of the hospitals in the total urban hospital review were Kaiser Permanente hospitals.

In total, they recognized 52 of the 1,200 hospitals as being the "Top Hospitals" in America.

How did we do?

Eighteen of the 52 "Top" hospitals were us. One national news piece referred to the results as "Kaiser Permanente dominating the list."

We are less than one percent of all the eligible hospitals in America. We were less than four percent of the high-performing hospitals whose performance was actually measured. And we ended up as 34 percent of the 52 best hospital winners.

Our goal is to be the best hospital system in America. We want to have the safest, most patient-focused hospitals. When people entrust us with their lives and their care, we want to be the right place for them to be.

This recognition from the Leapfrog Group indicates that we are moving in the right direction.

So my letter this week celebrates all of the hard work that all of our care teams have done to create a level of care and a standard of care that is being recognized as an inspiration to other care sites in the country.

Really well done. It's a great path to be on.

Be well.

George

✽ ✽ ✽

Background Note: Other Blood Stream Infections Also Need to Be Reduced – We are Doing Very Good Work

An earlier set of letters in this book dealt with sepsis and pressure ulcers. We have had amazingly good performance and very high success levels in reducing both sepsis deaths and pressure ulcer crises, damage, and deaths in our hospitals. We have also put a significant amount of energy into the area of preventing and reducing hospital-acquired infections. We won the Leapfrog Group recognition, in part, because of our successes in all of those areas.

Hospital-acquired infections is a major problem for our entire country. More than 1.7 million Americans enter a hospital every year and get an infection they did not have on the day they were admitted to the hospital.

So how have we done?

We are continuously learning and continuously improving.

The next set of letters in this book were among a number of weekly letters that addressed bloodstream infections in our hospitals. Those letters celebrated the successes we have had in bringing down both the number of infections and the lives lost to those infections.

Saving lives is always a good thing to celebrate. You can get a sense of the progress we have made by our journey of improvement that we have been on by reading the string of letters.

This is another area where data is pure gold as a tool and continuous improvement needs key data points to save lives.

Celebrating Hospital Performance – January 4, 2008

Dear KP Colleagues,

Primary bloodstream infections are the eighth leading cause of death in the U.S. today, with up to one half of the infections occurring in ICUs.

There are, in fact, roughly 80,000 BSI's each year in American ICU's. They result in over 14,000 deaths.

Those BSI deaths are a tragedy. The infections, themselves, can be a major personal disaster for the patient who gets one. Pathogens in the bloodstream can lead to sepsis — where overwhelming infection invades the patient's bloodstream with toxin-producing bacteria.

Great pain and suffering can result.

Kidneys, liver, lungs and the central nervous system can all be impaired. For the patients with sepsis, it can be a horrible and terrifying experience — and, as I said earlier, at least 14,000 die.

Many of those bloodstream infections can be prevented. That's why I am writing about those infections in my weekly letter of celebration. Caregivers can very carefully and methodically take steps to prevent those infections from happening.

Kaiser Permanente is moving in that direction. We will continue down that path because our patients are what we are all about — and we have caregivers who know what to do to prevent those horrible infections from happening.

In their How to Prevent BSI Guide, the Institute for Healthcare Improvement (IHI) offers a national average rate for bloodstream infections in the ICU of 5.3 infections per "1,000 line days." Because we consistently take steps to prevent those infections, Kaiser Permanente hospitals are now at 1.5 infections per "1,000 line days."

We can do better.

Our best performing Kaiser Permanente medical center in Portland, Oregon, has not had one single infection in 24 months. Not one. That's two full years of doing care very, very well relative to bloodstream infections.

Please join with me in congratulating our caregivers at Kaiser Sunnyside Medical Center for that achievement.

That's not our only exceptional hospital performance level for BSI's.

Our hospitals in Manteca, Orange County, and Santa Rosa also have reported multiple months with no ICU bloodstream infections. Caring people are doing the right things with amazing and wonderful consistency — and we are making a real difference in patient's lives because we are performing so very well.

How are those results achieved? With great attention to detail and a reliably designed process which includes evidence based interventions such as use of full barrier precautions during line insertion, use of chlorhexidine antiseptic for insertion site cleansing prior to insertion and during central line dressing changes, hand hygiene prior to insertion and dressing changes, appropriate insertion site selection, antiseptic-impregnated central catheters and insertion site dressings, use of adhesive anchoring devices instead of sutures for central lines, and catheter hub cleaning during central line dressing changes. Very smart people on our care team created those protocols. They work.

That whole approach may seem like a lot of focus on detail. For patients not suffering from the terrors and agony of a bloodstream infection — those are the details of angels, the wonderful focused and consistent details of truly caring about the lives and the clinical status of the patients we serve.

We are, by the way, pioneers nationally and internationally in actually measuring "days since a BSI." We initiated that specific quality measure with the help of IHI. We hope it becomes a nationally embraced strategy for engaging patients and clinicians in efforts to further reduce infection risk for all hospitals. Patients' lives will be better if that happens.

So join with me in congratulating the heroes from our Northwest Region for showing us all — and the world — what can be done about BSI's and then actually doing it.

Be well — and welcome to 2008.

George

* * *

Celebrating Zero Infections – March 28, 2008

Dear KP Colleagues,

A couple of months ago in my weekly letter, I celebrated the fact that our hospital in Portland, Oregon, had managed to achieve over two years without a single bloodstream infection for a single patient.

Those infections can absolutely ruin a person's life. They are extremely painful and patients with those infections can end up with major organ dysfunction and even organ failure.

In fact, people die of those infections. The people who survive often need a lot of care for a very long time. Some are permanently damaged and never fully recover.

When hospitals take all of the proper precautions, and are very systematic in taking steps to avoid those infections, those infections become extremely rare and can even disappear entirely.

This is a relatively new learning for American health care. For many years, hospitals just assumed that those infections were "a fact of life" and would periodically just happen. We are now much smarter about those issues. We now know we can make a real difference.

So what am I celebrating this week? I am celebrating the fact that the Kaiser Permanente Sunnyside Hospital continues to be infection free. I am also celebrating the fact that Sunnyside has now been joined by six other Kaiser Permanente hospitals that have each gone over a year since they have had a single infection.

The six hospitals are: Panorama City, Manteca, San Francisco, Santa Rosa, South San Francisco and Vallejo.

Both California Regions now have hospitals that have gone over a year without a single bloodstream infection.

Those hospitals have systematically and vigorously put in place the basic processes and steps necessary to protect our patients from those infections.

Please join with me in saluting Panorama City, Manteca, San Francisco, Santa Rosa, South San Francisco and Vallejo, along with Kaiser Sunnyside, for their success.

Because of the excellent work done by the care teams at those hospitals, patients did not have to go through intensely miserable and life threatening experiences. The care teams at those hospitals cared enough to do some very basic things consistently right.

(You can go to IHI.org for a description of the approaches used to reduce or eliminate infections.)

The rest of our hospitals have also significantly reduced their infection rates. Our overall numbers for our own hospitals are better than the national averages now and our hospitals are getting even better. For seven of our hospitals, we now are tied for being the very best in the world... infection free for over a year. Number one is a very good place to be when patients' lives are at stake.

Be well,

George

✿ ✿ ✿

Celebrating Systematic Care Improvement – September 12, 2008

Dear KP Colleagues,

Roughly one year ago, I wrote a weekly celebration letter that focused on the excellent progress our Northern California hospitals had made relative to both hospital infection rates and levels of pneumonia acquired prior to hospitalization.

I celebrated our systematic focus on doing the right things at the right time for our hospital patients, and I included a chart showing the huge levels of improvement that had happened in those hospitals.

I also celebrated — a bit later in the year — the fact that four of our hospitals had each gone a full year without one single infection.

Those infections can do so much damage to a patient that we all ought to appreciate what a huge achievement it was for those four hospitals to go a full year without one single infection.

At the time I wrote those letters, our Southern California hospitals had also started down that path of systematic improvement. We were on track in that region and making great progress. I promised a letter on that topic later in the year.

So this week, I have a double celebration. The chart below shows our community acquired pneumonia results for our Southern California hospitals. Every single hospital in Southern California now has better results than our best hospital in 2006.

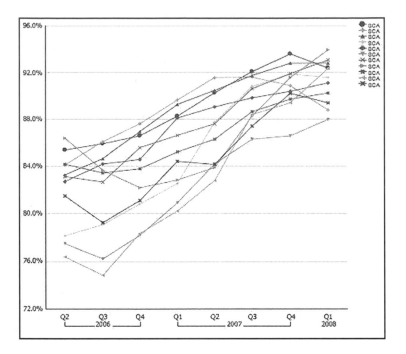

The definition of care measured by those charts is shown at the end of this letter.

This is still a work in progress — but major and measurable progress is being made.

Our goal is to have the very best hospital safety and quality scores in the entire country. If we work systematically — as a highly collaborative, patient-focused team of caregivers — we can achieve that result of being the very best.

I mentioned that there were two celebrations this week. The second celebration is an update on our initial success in totally avoiding all central line blood stream infections in a given hospital's ICU for more than twelve consecutive months.

When we originally celebrated that achievement, we had four hospitals performing at that level. That is already a top-quality "best" score because no other hospital in America can mathematically beat "zero" infections.

Today, I am very happy to report that we now have eight hospitals at that zero infection level and we have seven more hospitals that have had only one infection each in the past year.

The perfect-score for a whole year hospitals were Baldwin Park, Hayward, Orange County (Anaheim), Roseville, Santa Rosa, South Bay (Harbor City), Sunnyside (NW), and Vallejo.

The near-perfect hospitals were Bellflower, Fremont, Manteca, Redwood City, San Francisco, Santa Teresa (San Jose), and South Sacramento.

This is excellent care. It took a lot of work by dedicated caregivers who are going the extra mile every day to make life better for the patients we serve. We should all be proud of those results.

Years ago, hospital infection rates and community acquired pneumonia rates were not even measured. People died all the time from infections they should not have had — and no one did anything systematic to stop those infections from happening because no one even knew how many infections were happening.

Now that we know the numbers and we also know the science, we can make a difference. So we are making a difference.

Congratulations to all the folks who are making better care in our hospitals very real.

Be well.

George

* * *

The chart above measures hospital adherence to a composite of several best practices for pneumonia care. These practices include administering an antibiotic within a few hours of hospital arrival, giving flu and pneumococcal vaccines to at-risk patients, taking blood cultures prior to the administration of antibiotics, and counseling the patient on smoking cessation, if applicable. (Go to the QualityNet website [http://www.qualitynet.org/dcs/ContentServer?cid=1089815967023&pagename=Medqic percent2FMeasure percent2FMeasuresHome&parentName=Topic&level3=Measures&c=MQParents] for the exact measures.)

Celebrating Our Hospitals with No Infections for Two or More Years – July 30, 2010

Dear KP Colleagues,

When I have written in my weekly letters about our infection rates in our hospitals, I have talked about how horrible it can be for patients to end up with an infection they did not have on the day of admission to the hospital.

Those infections, in total, now are the number one cause of deaths in hospitals across America — killing more people than cancer or strokes.

That is horrible. And really sad.

We can do important things to reduce the number of those infections.

We can also do very important things to reduce the likelihood of death for the people who actually get those infections.

I will be celebrating our successes in some of those areas in the weeks ahead. And I will also share thoughts about some areas where we still have progress to make on our pathway to being the safest set of hospitals in America.

We are learning every day.

We just had a team of our most senior hospital leaders go to London to study some hospitals there that have made spectacular progress in some areas of patient infection prevention and safety.

Our Kaiser Permanente team in London learned that those hospitals were, in fact, spectacular in some important areas — and our team learned that we are actually doing better in some other safety areas.

The two care teams ended up teaching each other. That's a good place to be. Shared learning is one of the best ways to learn.

But that's not my celebration for this week.

What I am celebrating this week are some successes we are having in bloodstream infection rates.

Earlier this year, I celebrated the fact that we were delivering safe care so well that we had nine hospitals that had gone over a year without a single bloodstream infection in their adult ICU. We also, at that point, had two Kaiser Permanente hospitals that had gone two full years without an infection.

We now have four Kaiser Permanente hospitals that have gone over two years without a single bloodstream infection in their adult ICU.

And we now have 10 hospitals who have each gone over a year without an infection in our adult ICUs.

One hospital — South Bay — got to 33 months without one single infection.

Then an infection happened. So South Bay is now back to a restart and is building a new string of successes.

I expect them to continue to be a safety leader, and I suspect they will regain the front levels of safety success because our folks in South Bay have made a team commitment to patient safety that will continue to create success.

This is important work.

Those can be very nasty infections.

When any of us have a person we love in the hospital — or when we are personally in the hospital — we very much want that hospital to be a safe place. Our members and patients who go to the hospital very much want that hospital to be a safe place.

We are committed to being that safe place.

So congratulations to Fresno, Manteca, Panorama City, and Riverside for two full years without one single ICU bloodstream infection.

Well done.

Be well.

George

* * *

Background Note: We Win a Number of Quality Measurements

We clearly are doing good work as a quality leader for caregiving organizations relative to key areas of patient safety.

We also tend to do well on other quality measures — particularly, quality of care areas that have been set up by outside organizations who measure and compare quality performance.

Some of my favorite weekly letters deal with our pure quality wins. We particularly like being rated number one. It's good to be the best care system in America for many NCQA HEDIS measurements. In many areas of HEDIS measurement, being the best in America nationally also means being the best in the world. On mammograms, for example, we probably do better than all other countries relative to our success levels. Other countries tend not to have national scorecards with these kinds of quality measurements.

I have talked to ministers of health from multiple countries who were impressed by our willingness as a country to measure quality in so many ways. Most other countries do not have an NCQA equivalent process. That is unfortunate for them.

In any case, we tend to do well on any standardized quality measurements.

We have been the top performers in the country in nearly two dozen HEDIS categories. We love being number one. The next several letters are typical weekly letters that I wrote to our care teams celebrating some of those national quality wins.

Celebrating Our Number One Mammography Rates – October 30, 2009

Dear KP Colleagues,

The American Cancer Society tells us that when breast cancer is detected in its earliest stages, the survival rate is 98 percent.

That's not as good as 100 percent — but it's a much higher survival rate than cancers that are not detected until their late stages.

We know that to be true — so we want to detect breast cancers as early as we can.

The best early detection technique is mammography. To detect breast cancer early, we need our members to have their mammograms.

We have set up programs across Kaiser Permanente to help women schedule and receive mammograms.

We have call-up programs, reminder programs, and aggressive, consistent, and persistent mammogram scheduling programs of one kind or another in every region. We are using KP HealthConnect®, our electronic medical record, to trigger reminders to our caregivers at every kind of visit that a patient is due or overdue for a mammogram. We have linked our medical record very directly and intentionally to our mammogram reminder process.

So how well is that working?

The national HEDIS quality scores for last year have just been released. We now know exactly how we are doing in every region relative to our mammography success.

We are number one.

Number one in the country and maybe number one in the world.

Our Hawaii Region now has the best score of any health plan in America. Our Hawaii Region has done a wonderful job of encouraging and helping women to get their mammograms.

Nearly 6,000 of the more than 30,000 Hawaii members who were scheduled for mammograms in 2008 signed up because of HealthConnect reminders. Those reminders were combined with consistent "in-reach" by our Hawaii caregivers when members came in for various unrelated appointments for things like colds and eye exams. We love that approach because it works. Our Hawaii caregiver team has already doubled our in-reach program through the first half of 2009 — and we could triple it before this year is up.

We even put a mammography machine on the new Kaiser Permanente mobile clinic mega van that now takes care from town to town on the Big Island. We expect that mobile clinic to add another 4,000 mammogram screenings next year to our Hawaii total.

But even before that mobile clinic starts doing on-site mammography, Hawaii is number one — with the very best HEDIS score in the country.

How did we do in our other regions? We did well.

We had the best scores of any health plan in every Kaiser Permanente region.

Northern California and Southern California both had better scores than any other California health plan — with scores 10 percent better than the plan right behind us.

Colorado was number one in that region — with about a four percentage point lead over the number two plan.

Georgia had a very high score that was nearly 15 points better than the number two local plan — and our Georgia Region had the third highest score of all health plans in America.

Mid-Atlantic was number one with local health plans as well — with a mammogram rate that was more than eight percentage points over the second place local plan.

Northwest also had the highest local score — nearly five percentage points higher than the second place plan.

And Ohio, our smallest region, had the best scores in that area — with another local plan very close behind but nearly three percentage points behind us.

So we had the best mammography scores in the nation and we also had the best scores in each local region.

Our goal is to do even better next year. We are on a path to do exactly that.

Early detection of breast cancer means that lives are saved — so we need to do what we can do to save lives.

So my letter this week is about saving lives and about making a real difference in a lot of people's lives.

Congratulations to the total care teams in Hawaii and Georgia for leading the nation in mammography rates — and congratulations to the teams in each Kaiser Permanente region who made us the best in each local area.

Being best is a good place to be — not because it's good to win, but because it's really good to do good — and it is true that a good measure of doing good in some things is to be the best.

Be well.

George

✿ ✿ ✿

Celebrating A Number One Health Screening Score For Women – December 4, 2009

Dear KP Colleagues,

Chlamydia can make women sterile. It can do permanent damage to the fallopian tubes, uterus, and surrounding tissues.

It also can lead to chronic pelvic pain — and pregnant women with Chlamydia are much more likely to have an ectopic pregnancy.

Women with Chlamydia are five times more likely to be infected with HIV, if exposed.

For most women, there are no symptoms.

So this damaging disease is not suspected — and therefore it is not detected in many women until serious damage has been done.

Early detection requires a care system that cares enough about women patients to make Chlamydia testing and detection both a priority and an active agenda.

That would be us.

We want to detect Chlamydia as soon as we can in order to cure it and keep women healthy.

We have made Chlamydia detection a priority across Kaiser Permanente.

How are we doing? HEDIS measures Chlamydia detection as one of its national standards. We know how well we are doing relative to the rest of America.

We have the best scores.

Georgia had the very best scores of any health plan in America.

We had seven of the top 10 scores in the entire country. Only our Northwest Region was not in the top 10 in the country and the Northwest has the highest scores in their geographic service area, and was in the top 10 percent of plans for the country.

How did we do so well? Systematically. Patient by patient. We made Chlamydia detection a priority and our caregivers at the front line encourage women to have those tests.

Our electronic medical record gives us an incredibly useful tool so we know who has and who has not had their tests. Combining our commitment to helping women detect and cure the disease with our systematic support of women's care put us in a position where we do a better job than almost anyone on Chlamydia detection.

More than one million American women will have Chlamydia this year. In far too many settings, detection of this disease will be slow — and in some cases it won't be detected and diagnosed at all. A lot of undetected damage is happening to a lot of women.

So what I am celebrating this week is our commitment to making sure that we help minimize that damage for the women we serve.

Georgia was number one in the country. Mid-Atlantic was number two. Colorado was number three. Southern California was number four. Northern California was number six. Hawaii was number seven. And Ohio was number nine.

HEDIS measures the performance of roughly 230 health plans. Being in the top 10 doesn't happen by accident. Smart people need to do smart things in a consistent way to get our care teams to those levels of success.

Congratulations to our caregivers who care enough to make a difference in so many women's lives.

Be well.

George

* * *

Celebrating Continuously Improving Care for Our Senior Members - April 1, 2011

Dear KP Colleagues,

Southern California is number one in the country on medical attention for Nephropathy.

The National Committee for Quality Assurance (NCQA) national reporting system for health plans scores over a thousand health plans on multiple quality measures. Nephropathy care is a high priority measure because kidney failure does such horrible things to patient's lives and focusing on how well care systems do for the care of those patients is an important thing to do.

The name at the top of the national list of all health plans is Kaiser Permanente.

Seven of our regions were number one in their region.

Colorado improved Nephropathy scores — and is now number two in the country.

Those scores do not happen by accident. Best care isn't something that just occurs. Smart and caring people need to work hard as teams in a focused way to be the best in the country.

Those were the scores for our commercial patients. For our Medicare patients, we were also number one in seven of our eight regions and Southern California again had the highest Nephropathy score in the country.

We do a great job for our Medicare Advantage patients — with some of the highest scores in the country for multiple levels of care quality for seniors.

If you have a parent or friend or family member who is Medicare eligible, it can be a good idea to suggest to them that joining Medicare Advantage with Kaiser Permanente can be a path to great care. As I have said before, I wish my own mother lived in a Kaiser Permanente region so I could have the peace of mind of knowing she was a KP Medicare Advantage member.

I suspect I could persuade her to enroll. It would be a joy to be able to do that. Team care is particularly good when you are old enough to need team care much of the time.

Doing a good job for our patients takes a team of people working together as a team... supported by systems and supported by timely reminders that the right care is needed. Team care from caring people is the winning approach.

So, my letter this week celebrates Southern California for doing a super job on the Nephropathy performance levels and roaring into first place for the entire country on the care of both "commercial" and Medicare patients, and all of our care teams who are giving great care to our members in so many places every day. It's the right thing to do.

Well done.

Be well.

George

☆ ☆ ☆

Celebrating Our Success in Hypertension Control – June 10, 2011

Dear KP Colleagues,

Hypertension affects 65 million American adults over age 18.

That's a lot of people with a significant health problem.

What's worse is the fact that more than half of the people with hypertension in this country have badly controlled blood pressure.

That's a bad thing for America.

Why is badly controlled blood pressure a problem?

Poorly controlled hypertension leads to heart attacks and strokes.

Hypertension kills.

The care system of this country currently fails most hypertensive patients.

The control success rate last year was only 46.6 percent for the total population of hypertensive patients in America.

That's less than half succeeding.

So how did we do at KP?

We did a lot better.

Team care makes a big difference.

We have teams of nurses, therapists, physicians, pharmacists, and nutritionists focusing on helping our members with hypertension do well.

Our teams do direct diagnosis, active intervention, and provide continued, structured, patient-focused care.

We don't just wait for hypertensive patients to show up in the office.

We have a registry of patients with hypertension that serves to identify at-risk patients.

And we periodically reach out to our patients instead of just waiting for patients to show up in our care sites with the damage that hypertension can cause.

We use evidence-based clinical solutions.

We use our electronic medical record to track our care and help our care teams remember to do the right care for each patient.

One brilliant thing we do is combine the two most effective hypertension drugs into one pill.

Why is that brilliant?

It is brilliant because our goal is to make the right thing easy to do — and taking one pill at one time is easier than getting and taking multiple pills.

One pill is significantly better than two for helping people consistently take their medication.

So how well does that entire KP intervention and prevention strategy work?

We just published a paper showing blood pressure control for all of our hypertension patients in Northern California.

We have identified more than 600,000 hypertensive patients in Northern California.

A chart using data from that paper is shown below.

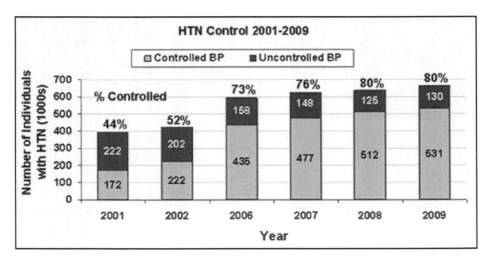

The rest of the country has fewer than 50 percent of hypertensive patients with controlled levels of the disease.

We used to be there as well.

We were at 44 percent in 2001.

We are now at 80 percent controlled.

Eighty percent is a big number.

Again — lives are being saved because we are doing the right thing for patients.

Organized, coordinated, process-supported, science-based care works.

We are doing the right thing, and we are doing it really well.

The Wall Street Journal featured our work.

A headline for the Wall Street Journal last week said "A Long-Awaited Advance in the War on Blood Pressure."

Here is a link to that article.

More than 250 other news outlets also ran and published stories about our success with hypertension patients.

The world now has a new standard for better hypertension care.

So my letter this week celebrates our care teams who have achieved 80 percent blood pressure control rates.

Really well done.

Be well.

George

✿ ✿ ✿

Celebrating Our Winning Cholesterol Management Scores – April 29, 2011

Dear KP Colleagues,

The number one key modifiable risk factor for cardiovascular disease and stroke — and the number two modifiable risk factor for diabetics — is lipid levels — cholesterol.

If we really want people to be healthier, the two most effective and consistent things that we can do for nonsmokers are to help people keep their cholesterol levels down and to help people who are inactive to consistently and regularly walk.

For smokers, the most effective thing we can do is to help people stop smoking. That's a topic for another week.

Walking helps people in multiple ways. Walking helps create better health. Go to our walking website for a wide range of solid information about activity levels and walking.

Walking doesn't have a HEDIS quality of care score yet. But cholesterol management does.

We know how well we do on cholesterol management compared to other health care organizations.

Over 250 health plans were measured last year by NCQA based on their ability to manage cholesterol levels for their cardiovascular patients.

How did we do on that national quality of care performance scale?

We were number one in the country — we were also number one in six of our regions, and we were number two in the other two regions.

The name at the very top of the national Medicare cholesterol performance chart was our Northwest Region.

Why is that performance level important?

People's lives are better when cholesterol is managed — because people with the right cholesterol levels have fewer strokes and fewer heart attacks.

We use both KP HealthConnect® and team care to achieve those number one scores. We have built focused and targeted decision support tools that are used by our caregivers in the exam room with the patient and — to make the right thing easy to do — we have one-click generators of the appropriate medical orders on our system, so doctors can order both tests and medications very easily.

One-click is the right number of clicks.

We win with team care — with nurses, medical assistants, nutritionists, pharmacists, and physicians all working together on patient-focused care teams to deliver best care to our patients.

Our computer systems provide a range of reminders for both caregivers and patients — and we scan our computerized database for members who have not been screened, have not been treated, or who have actually been treated and then discontinued their meds — so we know who currently needs our support for their care.

Bringing down cholesterol levels is the right thing to do. Doing it at the highest performance levels in the country is also the right thing to do.

This is a topic near and dear to my own health and heart. My own LDL levels used to be well past 150. Now — with a statin, some basic support, and eating almost no animal fat, zero cheese, no butter, and absolutely no red meat — I have dropped my own LDL count under 60, and I have kept it at that low level for over three years.

So I know personally that getting cholesterol to much lower and healthier levels can be done. It did not happen for me by accident. Some food items simply disappeared entirely and completely from my diet. But vegetables, fruit, grains, fish, chicken, and tofu in various forms are there in quantity — and my personal cholesterol levels now run much closer to where I want and need them to be.

So I feel particularly good about the fact that Kaiser Permanente now leads the entire country on that HEDIS cholesterol score.

My letter this week celebrates our teams of caregivers who work with our patients every single day to make us number one in the country for cholesterol scores.

Well done.

Be well.

George

* * *

Celebrating Our Quality and Service Wins – September 30, 2011

Dear KP Colleagues,

There is a national rating system for health plans in America.

NCQA — the National Committee for Quality Assurance — runs the rating system. NCQA looks at about 50 separate measures of plan quality, plan service levels, and plan infrastructure and processes to rate health plans.

In total, more than 1,000 plans across the country receive NCQA ratings.

I have written in earlier weekly letters about specific areas of health care quality wins for Kaiser Permanente. The NCQA Healthcare Effectiveness Data and Information Set (HEDIS) program measures and recognizes health plans in specific quality categories. Kaiser Permanente has had the highest quality scores in the country in a couple dozen HEDIS categories for both our Medicare patients and for our commercial health plan members.

We want to have the best and safest hospitals, and we want to deliver the best care in America — and in the world — so those individual category HEDIS wins are exactly the right direction for us.

NCQA does more than just measure individual quality scores.

NCQA also calculates a macro score for each plan and issues a total national ranking for all health plans. The total macro ranking of plans includes quality scores, service scores, and an evaluation of key health plan processes and infrastructure capabilities.

We have had a series of national wins on our quality scores, and our infrastructure is always highly rated.

Over the past couple of years, we have been applying some of the same energy and skills to our service levels that we have always dedicated to our quality levels.

How is that additional focus on service going?

It is going well.

Our new total NCQA scores have just been announced. The combined scores look good. Very good.

For our "commercial" members, our total quality and service rankings are the highest of all local plans in six of our regions. Our six largest regions each have total melded service and quality scores for our commercial members that win locally and also rank in the top 10 percent of all plans for the country. Our two smallest regions are in the top 20 percent for "commercial" members for all plans in America.

Those were our "commercial" patient rankings.

So how did we do in the national rankings for our Medicare patients?

We won.

Our KP Medicare Advantage plans swept the top four positions in the country.

Four of the top five plans in the country for Medicare are us. Northern California was number one in the country. Southern California was number two. Colorado — number two in the country last year — is now number three — with even better scores than a year ago. Our Northwest plan was number four.

If this were the Olympics, every winner on the medal platform would be us.

Hawaii is now ranked number seven for the whole country. That's also a great score.

Our other smaller regions each had the highest Medicare rating in their local market area. Each scored in the top 10 percent of all Medicare plans for the entire country.

Those ratings are really good news. Our service levels and care quality affect a lot of people. We have a million Medicare patients and members. A million is a big number. We want to be the best place in the country for people on Medicare to get care. Being the best is our goal.

The new NCQA Medicare ratings indicate that we are on the path to achieve that goal.

Earlier this year, J.D. Power and Associates — the global research company — released their own regional ratings of health plan satisfaction levels. J.D. Power rates health plans across the country, as well. They also rate cars, phones, power companies, drug stores, and multiple other businesses and industries. You often see J.D. Power ratings mentioned in ads for the winners.

How did we do on their rating scorecard for employer satisfaction with health plans?

We won there, also.

KP just won the top J.D. Power rating — with a number one ranking on service for KP as a health plan in five regions.

J.D. Power and NCQA aren't the only organizations who rate health plans. A company called "Satmetrix" also does its own national ratings — measuring customer loyalty levels for companies in various industries. The "Satmetrix" people survey customers about various products, and then they rate the companies by the comparative level of customer brand loyalty.

So how did we do on the "Satmetrix" national customer loyalty level rating for major health plans?

We won.

We not only won, we had scores that ran far higher than the average scores of other large health plans.

It's a very good thing when our members feel loyalty to us. Loyalty has to be earned. It is not just awarded.

We care deeply about our members. Great quality and great care comes from deeply caring about each member. Quality improvement isn't easy. Best care and safe care are both constant commitments. It's work we do every single day, over and over, to make sure our patients get great care.

Service is a matter of both caring and respect. Respect is the key to great service.

Why?

Service comes from respecting our members enough to make our members' lives better. We win on service by doing the right things to make each of our members' lives easier and by meeting the needs of each member as a person.

It's sad to say, but some care systems are rude and discourteous and disrespectful of other people. It is extremely disrespectful at a very personal level to be rude or discourteous to a patient. It is also impersonally disrespectful when care organizations make patients' lives more difficult for purely administrative or bureaucratic reasons.

We have the exact opposite perspective. We appreciate and respect our members and our patients. It is extremely respectful to not only be courteous and cooperative and administratively competent — but to go the extra ten feet or even the extra mile when our members need us to go that extra distance.

I received an email about going the extra mile last Friday that came from a member. The member gave me permission to include his letter in my weekly letter to all of our folks. The letter from our member is about service. I have included it.

So what am I celebrating this week?

I am celebrating our absolutely great NCQA scores and rankings — and our J.D. Power scores — and our Satmetrix scores — and all of the people who made those top-level new national rankings real for KP and our members.

We should be proud of what these scores tell us about what we do for the people who entrust us with their lives and their care.

I am also celebrating the KP care team folks who reached out to the member who wrote the letter below and made the nice difference in his life. The special treatment didn't save his life. It made his life easier. His opening words in his email were — "Do I love Kaiser?"

I suspect you will like the answer.

Letter from KP Member
Do I love Kaiser?
Why, yes I do!
Before I left on a trip to Europe, I developed a sinus infection. Darn it!
So, how did Kaiser take care of me?
1. Did they offer an advice nurse who was readily available via phone? YES, THEY DID!
2. Did they offer me a telephone consult with a physician who had my medical record at her finger tips? YES, THEY DID!
3. Did they provide nearby, convenient pharmacy service even though I was at my Mother's house in the Bay Area and not my own in Davis? YES, THEY DID!
4. And was the facility clean, safe, secure and with plentiful parking? YES, IT WAS!
5. And was there minimal wait in line at the pharmacy? YES, IT WAS MINIMAL (MEASURED IN THE FOLLOWING MANNER: "LESS THAN A MINUTE IN LINE".)
6. And did ALL OF THIS happen on a national holiday? WHY, YES, IT DID!

And was I able to quickly get in to see my primary care provider within 24 hours to make sure I was totally ready health care wise for an overseas vacation right after this holiday, given that I had just started this sinus infection?

The answer is: YOU BET!

And, so, I think the answer to the question in the subject line, "Do I love Kaiser?" should be obvious by now.

And, there is not a single word of exaggeration here. Kaiser folks were terrific, including the ones who had to listen to me hack over the telephone as the sinus infection was starting to eat me up.

The level of service was just breathtaking!

Thought you might want to know.

Regards,

John

Nicely done.

Be well.

George

✿ ✿ ✿

Background Note: People From Around the World Want to Learn from Us

We are somewhat unique in being both a fully functioning, vertically integrated care system and also, at the same time, a funder of health care — a health plan. We bring all of the pieces together. We get paid a premium every month to provide all care for each member rather than just being paid unit-price fees for individual pieces of care. That is a much better financial model when you want to achieve continuous improvement in care delivery.

It is good to be free from fees as a primary source of revenue. Most people who are not health care professionals do not understand how perverse and limiting the consequences of a purely traditional fee-based financing model and cash flow can be. Fees literally dictate care delivery in most care settings in this country. Most American care sites only do the care pieces and the specific care procedures that are listed on an approved insurance company fee schedule. That limitation of practice creates real rigidity for care delivery that can sometimes endanger patients, and it directly penalizes any process re-engineering.

Because we aren't fee-based at Kaiser Permanente, we can focus on actual patient care needs rather than limiting our approaches to specific pieces of care that we can submit as bills to an outside insurer to receive individual medical claims payments. We aren't limited to that fee schedule to define our care, so we can invest very differently in the infrastructure of care, the process of care, and in the care support tools we use.

As an example, 14 of the things we do to cut the HIV death rate in half do not show up on a Medicare or insurance company fee schedule. The death rate could double if we stopped doing those things.

Our fee-free financial model — selling care by the package and not by the piece — fascinates people from many countries. Kaiser Permanente is studied by both health systems and by the governments of other countries. We actually function a lot like a country. We have a single macro-budget, and we provide a full spectrum of care to a defined population of patients. Other countries see that we have really great outcomes and results.

As noted earlier, we are responsible for the total care of our covered population of nine million people. And we do it to scale. We aren't a little experimental pilot site somewhere. We are actually bigger as a care system than 42 states and 135 countries. Other countries see that we have better team care and much better care systems and more complete care support infrastructure than almost anyone else in care.

So we constantly have a stream of visitors from around the world who come to visit us to see what we do. We are also on a lot of agendas for international care meetings and conferences.

One thing that makes us very relevant to other countries is that people in other countries also have chronic conditions as their number one cost driver. Other countries are also implementing electronic medical records for their care sites, and those other countries very much want to figure out how to use those tools to improve care, particularly for their chronic care patients with co-morbidities.

So a lot of other countries are facing the same issues that we are trying to resolve — and many want to learn from us.

That's good, because we do love to teach.

The next four letters celebrate our teaching role for people from several other countries.

It's good to be able to help.

Celebrating The Global Health Policy Summit – August 10, 2012

Dear KP Colleagues,

It was an interesting week last week at The Global Health Policy Summit in London.

Caregivers, government officials, and policy leaders from multiple countries came together to talk about the issues of health care delivery. A major focus of the summit was how to use computer support to improve care and make care safer.

Our program to cut HIV deaths to half of the national average was in the spotlight, along with the incredible research that we did to identify the impact of statins in improving survival levels for hospitalized stroke patients.

It was pointed out that we may be really the only health care database on the planet right now that could look at all of the stroke cases across a population of millions of patients and figure out what some key factors are for patient survival.

A senior operating officer of the British National Health Service (NHS) was very complimentary of our work and said that the next generation of care delivery in the United Kingdom would be modeled, in part, on what we are doing at Kaiser Permanente.

One of the fascinating discussions at the summit dealt with the fact that care delivery of the future will probably happen in four basic sites — Site One will be hospitals and their equivalents. Site Two will be clinics and their equivalents. Site Three will be the home. And Site Four will be the Internet — with diagnostic, therapeutic and care delivery work being done remotely with an amazing array of tools for a lot of people.

Some developing countries who can't afford to build robust care sites will rely on the fourth site of care very heavily to distribute knowledge to their various hinterlands — medically underserved geographies in those countries.

When you look at the four sites of care, we are clearly pioneering computer-supported care in all four sites.

That's good — because the future is less likely to damage us, derail us, and threaten us if we help invent it.

So we are thinking hard about how to deliver the right care in all sites. Quite a few other care systems around the world are impressed with where we are already.

One product of the summit was a report about future models and sites of care. The Digital Dimension of Healthcare Report (pdf), not coincidentally, mentions some of our KP achievements.

We are different from many of the organizations at the conference, because we are first and foremost a provider of care — and we build our tools to serve patients. That makes us very practical and functional in our thinking.

So my letter this week celebrates all of our care delivery teams and our care tool development teams who have gotten us so far down the road toward future sites of care.

We just released a press release this week saying that we lead the world in patient connectivity — with more than 4 million of our members now using our electronic tools. No one else comes close to kp.org in terms of functionality or use levels.

This week's letter celebrates all of the folks at KP who made that press release about our connectivity and The Global Health Policy Summit connectivity report possible.

Well done.

Be well.

George

✿ ✿ ✿

Celebrating KP International – January 11, 2008

Dear KP Colleagues,

An hour ago, I was in our board room in Oakland talking to health care leaders from twenty countries. They were here to meet with key members of our KP medical leadership team about how we are systemizing care support. They were also here to learn about our KP HealthConnect® agenda.

Over the past several years, we have had a steady stream of visitors from abroad who want to see what we are doing and how we are doing it. The visitors have often been very senior people from other countries. We have, in fact, hosted the senior ministers of health from several European countries in just the last few months.

The minister of health from Germany not only brought her senior leadership team, but also members of the German news media into both our board room and into our care sites.

The gentleman who is the Performance Director for the full National Health Service in England is spending a year on site with us as a Commonwealth Fund Harkness Fellow. He speaks very highly of the experience.

Very senior caregivers and governmental leaders from multiple countries have spent time with our Colorado Region, California Regions, and our Mid Atlantic Region to look at our operations and our approaches.

I want to thank the Kaiser Permanente caregivers in all of those sites who have been so generous with your time and expertise for all of those visits and all of those visitors. The foreign health care leaders love coming to real world care sites that actually coordinate care, focus on health, and use computers to support care. When they can visit and touch an actual care site and see real care, that is often far more valuable to our foreign visitors than reading an article, hearing a speech, or attending a seminar.

Kaiser Permanente folks also have spoken at a number of international seminars and conferences, both in the U.S. and abroad. Several Kaiser Permanente senior physicians and leaders have spent significant time in Britain with the National Health Service. We have also had physicians and labor leaders visit European care sites, both to learn and to teach.

I had the honor and pleasure a couple of years ago of being invited to attend a meeting of European Union Health Ministers in Chantilly, France. Because Kaiser Permanente is so large — larger than several European Union countries — and because we have a fully integrated care system with a responsibility for population health, they granted me honorary status as a working "health minister" and allowed me to attend the off-the-record, private "health minister only" meetings. It was fascinating to hear the health ministers from countries like Norway, Switzerland and the Netherlands discuss their agendas, challenges and problems. They asked me to chair the last three hours of the final meeting — when the originally-designated chair of the meeting had to return to his home country, ahead of schedule.

I can tell you for a personal fact that the rest of the world cares about what we are doing and is closely watching what we are doing. Dr. Jack Cochran, our new head of The Permanente Federation, was just asked to address a major meeting of British medical leaders in England and he spent quality time with Lord Darzi — the Minister of Health for that huge health system — talking about the common issues we face and the solutions we are developing.

On the one hand, that is all very complimentary to Kaiser Permanente. On the other hand, it really is an accountability for us at this point in our history.

We are looked at so closely by people from those countries because we have the knowledge base, organizational model, patient accountability, and delivery system that others want to understand and — in many areas — emulate.

So we are sharing. We are hosting tours of our sites and we are teaching folks in their sites. The rest of health care needs us to be a resource — not just here, but for the world.

So this week I am celebrating our small international staff in Oakland who supports that flow of people into our learning sites, and I am celebrating and thanking all of our caregivers who take time from your busy lives to hold the hands and channel the learning for all of those foreign folks who came here to visit us and learn.

It takes time. It takes extra effort. It is above and beyond the call of duty. It is really well done. It helps people across the planet get a sense

of the value we are creating at Kaiser Permanente. I thank you for taking the time, extending the welcome, and for being great hosts.
Be well.
George

✿ ✿ ✿

Celebrating International Learning – November 19, 2010

Dear KP Colleagues,

We are holding a meeting of the Board of Directors for the International Federation of Health Plans near San Francisco today.

The International Federation has more than 100 member health plans from 30 countries.

Most people think that health plans do not exist in countries that have universal coverage. In truth, every country with universal coverage has competing private health plans. Only Canada doesn't have full-scale health plans — and even in Canada, there are a couple of small health plans that exist because six of the eight Canadian provinces don't cover prescription drugs for their citizens — so people in those provinces buy private coverage for their pharmaceutical expenses.

Two of the Canadian plans are at the meeting today.

Why are all of those health plans meeting here?

They are here to look at our automated medical record, our care management programs, and our computer support functionality.

They are here to learn from us.

They also are here to teach. Every country does several things very well — and these meetings give us all a chance to share best practices — and to share and discuss problems, issues, and challenges.

Every single country is facing its own health care cost crisis.

Sharing our thinking and our approaches is an enjoyable thing to do.

The health plans who are here today join a long list of foreign visitors who have visited us this year.

We also have had some pretty senior visitors come to KP.

The ministers of health from Denmark and Switzerland both brought teams of their people to study us this year.

You can link to a fun translation from a Danish newspaper report about the visit their health minister had here.

We have had half a dozen other ministers of health visit us over the past couple of years.

We have had actual delegations from Belgium, Canada, Ireland, the Netherlands, New Zealand, Norway, Singapore, Switzerland, and the United Kingdom visit us this year. Each of those countries had a team of people who attended a customized teaching session presented by our KP caregivers and our systems team.

We also had folks come to study us from Brazil, China, Colombia, the Czech Republic, the Dominican Republic, Estonia, Finland, Germany, Hong Kong, India, Israel, Mexico, Nigeria, Pakistan, Peru, the Philippines, Qatar, Spain, South Africa, Sweden, Taiwan, the United Arab Emirates, and Zimbabwe.

I have had a chance to meet with a number of our visitors.

They really like seeing the fact that we can actually deliver team care in a patient focused way — and we can use our computers to support our caregivers rather than just generate bills.

Today, at our International Federation board meeting, the visitors are looking at our systems. They also are here to learn about the current overall status of health care reform in America.

Conversations have been animated. Questions have been pointed and well thought through.

We have a great chance to help this country get reform right.

Every time I meet with our visitors from other countries, I am reminded of what we have accomplished and of all the important things we have yet to do.

We are on a path. We are part way down that path. It's a good path to be on, but we need to keep ourselves in a momentum of continuous improvement to where we need to be.

Teaching is often a great way to learn.

Explaining where we are to other people can sometimes be a very useful part of figuring out exactly where we are.

So my letter this week celebrates all of the people who come to Kaiser Permanente to learn — and also celebrates all the people who share with us the good things they have already learned.

Learning is a good place to be and a good thing to do.

Be well.

George

✳ ✳ ✳

Celebrating 27 Mentions of Kaiser Permanente – April 13, 2012

Dear KP Colleagues,

Sixty health plans from 40 countries met in Argentina last month to share learnings with each other about health care delivery and health care financing.

A well-known national health care consultant from the U.S. who attended the conference told me that he noticed that Kaiser Permanente was mentioned in the very first talk, so he decided to keep track of how many times KP was referenced by various speakers at the conference.

He made a tic list on his printed agenda for the conference. At the end of the conference, he counted 27 mentions of Kaiser Permanente. We were referenced 27 times by various speakers at that highly international meeting.

That list of mentions doesn't include one of our own senior medical leaders who did a third-day keynote talk for the meeting where he explained to the attendees our vision and our strategy at KP for the future use of health care delivery support tools and computerized care information resources.

That session about KP's vision and strategy clearly impressed people. It was not, however, the only session at the conference that featured intelligent and skillful use of computerized data resources and innovative connectivity approaches.

One of the speakers from a relatively new and surprisingly large health plan from Eastern Europe explained that his organization is now using a blend of home-grown electronic medical records, patient-focused electronic disease registries, and email connections with patients to echo and almost clone in some respects what we are doing with those same tools.

That speaker from Eastern Europe said their team had directly used KP as a model and an inspiration and a teacher for their work and for parts of their organizational approach.

The Eastern European plan is doing some very good things and they seem to be doing them well. People are benefitting from their care.

I talked to a seasoned health care leader from Great Britain who attended the conference. He said, "Kaiser Permanente is dragging the rest of health care into this century." He seemed pleased.

We are far from perfect. We are very much learning as we go. Our own systems are in a state of continuous improvement rather than being in a state of final development ... but we really are doing some very important work in a number of key areas.

I wrote a letter three weeks ago about the nominees for the Vohs Award for Quality at Kaiser Permanente. More than half of the 15 nominees for that quality award used our new electronic health record tool kit in very innovative ways to make care better.

We will continue to be on the international stage. Next month, the Healthcare Information and Management Systems Society (HIMSS) of Europe will meet in Copenhagen, Denmark.

That meeting will be a lot smaller than the HIMSS USA meeting in February that attracted 37,000 people.

We had several speakers at the HIMSS USA conference last month — and we won their Davies Award for organizational excellence in the use of IT to support care.

In Europe, we won't win any awards but the HIMSS conference in Copenhagen will basically have a Kaiser Permanente morning featuring a keynote speech about KP followed by several sessions involving Ministers of Health from European countries who will — in part — be discussing what KP is now doing.

That is next month. In two months, more than 30 chief information officers from around the world will come to a special meeting in Oakland to spend a couple of days learning from our IT leaders and our health care leadership, our agenda, and our successes.

People who have signed up for that session tell me they are very excited about the chance to use us as a model for figuring out their own future.

We sometimes say that the world is noticing what we do ... and it is clear that is very true.

What makes us special and worth watching is that we are not just academic or theoretical or hypothetical or even philosophical in our teachings and our learnings. We are extremely practical. We are grounded in the day-to-day reality of patient care and also grounded every single day in the reality that we are responsible for the health and care for an entire population.

We have both the ability and the reason to use systems and resources and knowledge in a way that very few other more splintered care sites can do. Our total agenda makes us a model for the world. But being a model for the world isn't why we do what we are doing. Better patient care is our goal. Getting care right for the people we serve is our goal. Making the right thing easy to do for our caregivers and our patients is our goal. That's who we are.

If others can benefit from what we learn as we focus on being who we are, that's good for the world, and it is one important way that we add value to the world around us.

So my letter this week celebrates us as a learning organization — a team of folks on a path of continuous improvement — and it celebrates the fact that we are very willing and more than happy to help the rest of the patients and the rest of the caregivers of the entire world benefit from what we learn.

It was nice to hear from the expert that speakers from other countries at the conference last month mentioned us as an example in their talks 27 different times in three days.

We seem to be helping.

Well done.

Be well.

George

☆ ☆ ☆

Background Note: Diversity is One of Our Major Strengths

A frequent subject of my celebration letters is our wonderful diversity. In fact, the very first letter that I wrote to our employees ten years ago right after I had joined Kaiser Permanente expressed my personal strong beliefs about diversity. I wrote in that very first letter to all members of the KP team a decade ago that diversity is and will be one of our major strengths. We are wonderfully diverse. We love being diverse. The next couple of letters make that point. Kaiser Permanente is one of the most diverse care systems in America and maybe on the planet. We have diverse caregivers, diverse staff members, diverse leadership, diverse membership, and diverse patients. We deliver care in some of the most diverse parts of our country. We believe that our diversity creates a synergy, a connectivity, and a rich and robust creativity that is key to much of our success. We win a lot of quality and service awards as an organization. I believe we earn those awards in part because our diversity helps us focus on all of our patients and not just on a subset of our patients who fit some stereotype of who a patient "should" be.

I also believe we perform at such a high level because we are clearly a meritocracy. In too many work settings, employees believe that promotions, advancement, and recognition go disproportionately to some subset of the work force. That obviously isn't true for us — as the next letters point out. So high performers from every segment of our population know that high performance is our agenda and not favoritism of any kind.

That creates a whole different work environment.

The following letters all celebrated our diversity. They were fun to write.

Celebrating Our Diversity Recognition – March 18, 2011

Dear KP Colleagues,

One of our greatest strengths is our diversity.

Kaiser Permanente is wonderfully diverse. We look today like all of America will look in another decade.

We have a diverse staff, a diverse membership, and a highly diverse governance process.

I have celebrated our diversity before. I have written about the fact that the KP Hospitals and Health Plan Board of Directors is less than 40 percent white male — in a world where boards of other organizations our size tend to be more than 80 percent white and more than 80 percent male.

Our workforce is 57 percent minority. We serve members in some of the most diverse cities in America — Honolulu, San Francisco, San Diego, Washington, D.C., Baltimore, Maryland, and Cleveland, Ohio.

We are an extremely high-performing care system. Our diverse teams of caregivers have put us in position to now have 23 separate HEDIS scores where the highest quality health plan in America is Kaiser Permanente.

We have won awards that no one else in health care has won for the dependability of our computer infrastructure — and we have been awarded 35 of the top 55 awards in the country for our hospital computerization levels. We dominate the Healthcare Information and Management Systems Society (HIMSS) Stage 7 awards.

We have the best computerized medical support tools in the world, and we are working to track care delivery by race, ethnicity, language, and gender to continually improve our ability to deliver the right care to all the segments of our patient population.

We have won awards for being a good place to work for LGBT workers, for African-American workers, for Hispanic women, and — at the end of the month — we will receive an award in New York City for being one of the best places to work for executive women.

Our CFO will be at the New York meeting giving a speech before we accept the award. She will be a highlight of their day of learning.

That is not what I am celebrating today.

DiversityInc magazine does an annual review of the 500 leading organizations in America, looking to see which companies are the best place to work for a diverse workforce.

We made the top 50 on that list three years ago.

We made the top five on that list last year.

This year, we won.

DiversityInc magazine just voted us number one as the organization in America that best reflected the right set of values and performance as an employer and worksite.

Sodexo won last year. Johnson & Johnson won the year before. Verizon Communications won the year before that. Bank of America won four years ago.

This year, the name at the top of the list is Kaiser Permanente.

That's a good place to be.

We are far from perfect. We are learning as we go. We make mistakes. We are sometimes clumsy, and sometimes go down paths that we need to correct.

Winning this award does not mean that we can say that we have nailed it — that we are as good as we can be.

Winning this award means that we are doing a lot of things right. Winning this award means we don't have a glass ceiling and we don't have institutionalized discriminatory practices and that we are eager to be inclusive and a great place for a very diverse population to work.

We are, as the people of Kaiser Permanente, committed to all of our patients from all of our diverse populations — and we are committed to being a team with ourselves to deliver great care.

We are far from perfect — but we are trying to do the right things and we are trying to do them for the right reasons.

For now, I want to celebrate all of the people at Kaiser Permanente who are so wonderfully effective and collectively caring that we can be a leader in so many ways we deliver care.

Our diversity is one of the reasons we do so well in so many areas.

This level of creativity could never happen in a world of pure clones.

We are smarter and we are better because we are so diverse and we benefit from our diversity.

DIVERSITY IS ONE OF OUR MAJOR STRENGTHS

So thank you to everyone who makes us being diverse so successful. We are learning and, as I said, we are not perfect — but we are definitely directionally correct.

That's a good place to be.

Be well.

George

✿ ✿ ✿

Celebrating Our Diversity – October 19, 2007

Dear KP Colleagues,

This week I am celebrating our diversity. Kaiser Permanente is one of the most diverse health care organizations in the world. We look today like the rest of America will look like in 20 years.

We have a very diverse employee base—with over half of our staff coming from one minority group or another. About 46 percent of our employees are Euro-American. That's less than half, so technically we don't even have a majority group inside of KP.

A number of other companies have very diverse staff at their very front lines—at the cash register or on the assembly line—but they have little or no diversity at the most senior levels of the organization.

That is absolutely not true of Kaiser Permanente. Take a look at the Website for the Kaiser Foundation Health Plan and Kaiser Foundation Hospitals Board of Directors. White males are a numerical minority on our Board. We have two Chinese-American Board members, two Latino Board members, three African-American Board members, five female members (three minority), and four white males.

We have one of the most distinguished, highly qualified, highly respected, and highly skilled Boards in America—current and former leaders of major American corporations and health care organizations. We very obviously do not have a KP glass ceiling that restricts our Board membership to Euro-American males.

So what about our senior management staff? A cynic might say, "You have an extraordinary Board—but what about the actual executives who are responsible for senior leadership? Are they all Euro-American males?

Nope. We have three executive vice presidents who make up our Operations Leadership Group. From the "OLG," our chief financial officer is a woman. One of our two senior operating officers is African-American, and the other is Euro-American. Very talented. Nicely diverse. The OLG has no glass ceiling.

We also, as you know, have eight Regional Presidents as the senior executive leadership for each of our eight health plans and our hospital systems. Over ninety percent of the health plan senior "president" level executives outside of Kaiser Permanente are white males. What does our team look like? We have six female presidents. Two of our presidents are Chinese-Americans. One is African-American. One is a white male.

Again—definitely not a glass ceiling.

We have received significant external recognition for our diversity. One organization named us a best place to work for Hispanic employees. Another named us a best place to work for Asian-American employees and another for African-American employees. The U.S. Department of Labor recognized us for our overall workplace diversity. Last month, we received a perfect score from the Human Rights Campaign as an employer of gay and lesbian employees.

You can read more about our awards on our National Diversity Website.

We have also been a leader in the areas of culturally competent care, and we have been a champion against racial and ethnic disparities in care. We have had multiple state, local, and national recognitions in all of these areas. This is work that needs to be done—and we are uniquely qualified and positioned to do it. So we are doing it.

Again, we are not perfect. We are human. We sometimes screw up, we make mistakes at times, and we are less than optimally sensitive at other times. We are a work in progress—but our goal is to be the very best as both a diversity employer and a multicultural caregiver.

"George C. Halvorson: It's time to give health care to all" Sacramento Bee, 09/14/07

In December, we will hold our thirtieth annual diversity conference. Over 1,000 of our caregivers, counselors, administrators, and workers will get together to study diversity, share best practices, discuss failures and shortcomings, and take steps to improve our ability to serve our increasingly diverse patient base. Ron Knox, our senior diversity leader, and his team have done spectacular work once again in putting together a great program of learning and sharing for that conference.

I would be surprised if any other caregiving institution in America can say they also go back thirty years on this same diversity-focused pathway.

Some people may remember that one of the very first letters I wrote to our staff when I got to KP was a letter about diversity. A copy of that letter can be found at the link below. I have been writing, talking, and learning about that topic for several decades. My next book is about diversity. My newest book has a chapter in it that deals with universal coverage as an issue of racial prejudice and ethnic disparity.

"Diversity, Done Well, Is a Clear Winner"George Halvorson, 09/1/03

So I personally love our magnificent diversity—and I have a sense we should all celebrate how wonderfully diverse we are. There is a great strength and beauty that comes from weaving a fabric from multiple threads. That's who we are and what we are doing.

I appreciate hearing from you. I am a little behind in my responses to feedback from earlier celebration letters, but I am reading them all. Thank you for writing.

Be well,
George

✿ ✿ ✿

Celebrating Being in a Diversity League of Our Own – May 25, 2012

Dear KP Colleagues,

One of our great strengths at Kaiser Permanente is our diversity.

We have a wonderful level of diversity among our caregivers and staff, and we have a wonderful level of diversity among our patients and members.

Our Board is diverse, our leadership is diverse, and our total array of caregivers is diverse enough that we don't have a majority group at Kaiser Permanente that makes up over half of our staff.

With the most diverse staff of any major health care organization, we perform at very high levels.

Medicare used 53 criteria to rate 459 health plans last year and gave their top plans five stars. Only nine health plans in the entire country were rated at five stars. Five of our regions rated the top level of five stars, and our lowest score in the other three regions was 4.5 stars.

We were also awarded the J.D. Power and Associates number one ranking for member satisfaction in our five largest Regions — and we have more than 20 HEDIS quality scores where the best score in the country is Kaiser Permanente.

So we are performing at high levels, and we are delivering care as teams in ways that save lives and set standards for others in health care.

My own strong opinion is that our diversity gives us the sensitivity and the connectivity that we need to serve our members respectfully and well.

Our commitment to our members and our patients, and our commitment to function in teams gives us performance levels that are what our members deserve because they entrust us with their care. That is a sacred trust, and one we appreciate.

So we do well when outside organizations rate us on quality and care. We also do well when outside organizations rate us relative to our diversity.

How well have we done?

We were rated number one in the country last year by DiversityInc's Top 50 Companies for Diversity as a best employer for diversity.

ComputerWorld magazine rated us the best place to work in the country for diverse IT employees. The people who give out the Catalyst Award as the best place to work for women gave us their first place award last year.

We have been recognized by the Hispanic College Fund as Company of the Year, and the National Hispanic Corporate Council will be honoring us at their annual meeting this year.

For the last two years, the Human Rights Campaign (HRC), the largest LGBT (Lesbian, Gay, Bisexual, and Transgender) advocacy group in the United States, recognized Kaiser Permanente for our fully inclusive, non-discrimination policy. We were named the first health and hospital system in the U.S. to earn a perfect rating, 100 percent, on the HRC's Health Equality Index. That means we were ranked the best health care system for LGBT.

Last year, Kaiser Permanente received a 90 percent rating on the HRC's annual Corporate Equality Index (Best place to work, for LGBT) for creating policies on diversity and inclusion, and providing training and benefits to create a fair and equal workplace.

One of my favorite awards comes from the Diversity MBA Magazine.

They rated us best employer in the country for diverse MBAs three years ago. Then they rated us again as number one as best employer in the country two years ago.

Last year, they rated us number one again.

It is a lovely thing for us to win first place three times in a row. That's good for us. But in an interesting way, it isn't quite as good for Diversity MBA Magazine to have the same winner year after year.

They throw a great banquet in Chicago every year for the winner.

They have a wide range of supportive organizations and diversity champions from across the country at the banquet. As the winner for the year, we are heavily featured at that dinner. We get to tell our story.

The attendees at the dinner were delighted and informed to hear our story the first year we won. They were reinforced and pleased to hear our story again the second year we won. They were — to be frank — slightly less excited to hear our story again for year three — even though we sent in a new team of very good presenters.

The winner each year goes on the cover of the magazine. Putting us on the cover three straight years probably didn't increase subscriptions.

Clearly, Diversity MBA Magazine had a problem.

So what did they do?

They came up with a lovely solution. They put us in a league of our own. They invented a new category of winner — Lifetime Achievement Hall of Fame Winner — and they made us the first organization to go into the Diversity MBA Magazine Hall of Fame. Three-time winners go into the Hall of Fame.

It's not unlike what happens in Europe for the winner of the Champions League each year in soccer. The winner of the Champions League each year gets promoted to the Premier League. That winning team then plays in the higher league the following year.

Diversity MBA Magazine promoted us to the Diversity Premier League, and they put us in the Hall of Fame. They still gave us a very nice recognition at the annual dinner, but they now get to name someone else as the annual winner, and the audience of the dinner now gets to hear how another organization champions diversity.

So that's what I am celebrating this week. I am celebrating being — for this one area of our performance — in a league of our own. Very cool.

Diversity is one of our greatest strengths and assets. We are far from perfect, and we will never get all of the issues right — but we are moving in some very good directions, and it is good to see those directions recognized.

Be well.

George

* * *

Background Note: Rosie the Riveter Was A Kaiser Employee

We come by our own diversity honestly. A commitment to diversity is not a new value for Kaiser Permanente. We have been diverse a very long time. Our cofounder, Henry J. Kaiser, owned shipyards in World War II that helped America win that war. Henry Kaiser had one of the first integrated work forces in the country at Kaiser industries — and he was the employer for the famous and iconic "Rosie the Riveter."

The new Rosie the Riveter National Museum is in Richmond — at the site of the old Kaiser shipyards. It's a lovely museum. Stop by and visit if you get a chance and you are in the Bay Area.

This weekly letter celebrated that history and that legacy.

I love the autographed poster of Rosie that hangs on my office wall.

Celebrating Rosie the Riveter, a Piece of Kaiser History – February 22, 2008

Dear KP Colleagues,

I just put a new framed and autographed poster on the wall of my office in Oakland. A reproduction of the poster is attached to the end of this letter.

The poster is one of the most famous posters ever done — "Rosie the Riveter" from World War Two. You will recognize it when you see it.

The poster was originally made to celebrate the fact that women in America were leaving their homes and going into factories to build the munitions, tanks, trucks and ships needed to defeat the fascist armies and navies allied against us.

Women did not work as welders in America before the war. Without women welders, there is a very good chance we would have lost the war. So the Rosie posters are important as a reminder of that success.

But why would I celebrate that poster and that point in history in my weekly celebration letter?

For starters, Rosie was one of us — a Kaiser employee and a Kaiser Permanente legacy patient. Henry Kaiser pioneered hiring women to work as welders and mechanics and electricians in the Kaiser shipyards at a point in time when women simply were not allowed to do that kind of work.

How well did that approach work? The Kaiser shipyards produced more ships than anyone ever dreamed possible. Before the war, the Nazi admirals had calculated how many ships their submarines would need to sink to cut Europe off from American supplies. The U-boats did their deadly job — but American ships continued to carry supplies across the ocean in very large part because the Kaiser shipyards got so good at building transport ships that they actually finished one boat in less than four days — from the point the keel was laid at the Kaiser shipyards in Richmond to the minute the ship steamed into San Francisco Bay under its own power.

Four days. Women welders at work.

I was attending an opening of a unit at our Richmond hospital a year ago and was asked by the hospital staff if I wanted to meet Rosie the Riveter. I was surprised and delighted. One of the original Rosies was at the hospital to attend the ceremony.

I had no idea that there were any surviving Rosies. I did know that I very much wanted an autographed Rosie poster. So I asked our communications team if we could sponsor a lunch for the Rosies who still live in the Richmond area to do just like the football and baseball stars do — sign their poster.

We had the lunch a few weeks ago and now I have a freshly autographed Rosie the Riveter poster hanging on my wall. I love it.

We had several posters signed — and we will be giving them as gifts to some appropriate recipients. I have no doubt that they will be treasured by the people who get them.

We did set two autographed posters aside to give as gifts to our staff in a drawing for the Kaiser Permanente folks who read this weekly letter from me and send an email asking to have your name put in the drawing for the posters. Tom Debley, our Kaiser Permanente historian, will be asked to draw the winning names in a week.

We have a great history. I am often amazed at how rich our total history as an organization is.

So my letter this week celebrates a piece of our history and it also celebrates my own very good fortune to now have a personally autographed Rosie the Riveter poster hanging on the wall in my office.

She looks great.

Be Well.

George

* * *

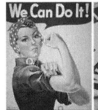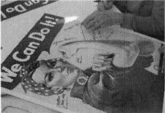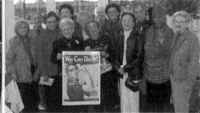

Background Note: We Are Also Working Hard to be Green

We need to be environmentally responsible.

My letters often celebrate our commitment at Kaiser Permanente to being environmentally responsible. As I keep saying in my letters, we clearly have only one planet. We need to be responsible stewards of the only planet we have.

As a health care organization, we had to learn to be green. That hasn't been a priority for many health care settings. It should be. We use a lot of energy and we use a lot of disposable materials. Many of the supplies and tools we use have to be disposed of in uniquely protective and safe ways. We generate millions of pounds of waste every year. We create environmental pressure at multiple levels.

So it is good for us to be environmentally sound in as many ways as we can.

The next several letters celebrate our commitment to being green. That commitment is very real — and it has been worth celebrating multiple times.

I am including several letters on being green in this book because they describe so many ways green can happen. Far too many health care sites and organizations do not make being green a priority — and I believe that happens because those sites do not know that green is possible. We are showing the world that green is possible, and I hope that sharing several letters on that topic might just be useful for other health care organizations who would like to be greener but don't know what specific green things can be done.

The letters also point to several categories of green awards. Health care organizations who want to be greener can contact those organizations to learn good ideas about being green.

These letters were very fun letters to write.

Celebrating Sharing Green – August 17, 2012

Dear KP Colleagues,

Three weeks ago, Kaiser Permanente was represented at the White House Council on Environmental Quality along with 10 other health care systems all committed to being environmentally responsible organizations.

About two years ago, we were a cofounder of the "Healthier Hospitals Initiative" — 11 health care systems with more than 500 hospitals who are all committed to using less energy, creating less waste, choosing safer chemicals, and serving healthier, sustainable food. That group was the foundation for the White House event.

Our own goal has been to be an environmentally safe and responsible care delivery organization.

We have been on this path for a number of years. Many of the elements included in the agenda for the new health care coalition are things we pioneered at Kaiser Permanente — including buying environmentally safe materials and using energy efficiently.

I have written about some of our green purchasing initiatives and our environmentally friendly building agendas in earlier letters.

One very recent achievement for us is that our Napa Data Center has now been rated as the only data center in the entire world to have platinum level certification by the Leadership in Energy and Environmental Design, for Existing Buildings, Operations and Maintenance (LEED-EB: O&M).

LEED is a certification awarded by the U.S. Green Building Council. The Building Council rates facilities and sites in multiple industries for environmental responsibility.

They give bronze, silver, and gold awards as well.

We won gold in the past. Now we are the first computer center in the world to win platinum.

What did we need to do to be graded as platinum?

We are doing some very good things in the design and operation of our computer center.

By managing our water consumption, we were able to cut our midsummer irrigation consumption by 95 percent, and we have reduced building water consumption by 48 percent. We even recycle the waste products from the site at a level that directs 66 percent of the waste away from going to a landfill. Our long term goal is 95 percent diversion of the waste.

You can't achieve those kinds of successes by accident or by pure goodwill. It isn't enough to wish we were green. We have some very smart people who are committed to being very green and who do very smart things to create that level of resource use.

Practice Greenhealth is another organization that gives awards to health sites for environmental excellence. They just rated us at a top level again. Over the past decade, we have won 142 awards from Practice Greenhealth.

Computerworld magazine also rates computer services across all industries for being relatively environmentally excellent. Only one health care organization made the Computerworld top 12 green-IT list for environmentally responsible computer organizations. We not only made the top 12 green-IT list — they rated us number one in the world.

I will probably write another letter later this year listing the amazing array of actual numbers that are involved and included in our total green agenda. We have done some important work and the overall numbers are impressive. It's another area where we need to measure performance in order to improve performance. Simply guessing about performance levels doesn't create great health care or great environmental protection.

It isn't enough just to be green, ourselves, however. It is clearly very important for us to be green. It is really the only responsible way for us to behave. But if we were to be the queen of green, and if everyone else outside of Kaiser Permanente continues to pollute and waste energy and use environmentally damaging chemicals — then the world will still suffer.

That's why we share what we do. We want a green world. That's why we created a really well-designed green purchasing formula checklist and then shared it with the world. That's why we share our strategies and our designs with others who also want to be green.

That's what I am celebrating this week. I am celebrating our sharing with 10 other health care organizations that took us to the White House to propose a set of achievable green goals for health care for the entire country. Nearly 100 news media outlets did stories about the White House event.

Our people have been key to that green health coalition effort. Our learning and our successes help reinforce the validity of the coalition's goals.

So our teams of people committed to being green here are also helping other people and other organizations to be green.

We only have this one planet. Let's take care of it.

So this week I am celebrating our green teams at Kaiser Permanente and the fact that our teams both learn and teach. We are far from perfect and we are learning as we go — but we are making a difference.

Well done.

Be well.

George

✿ ✿ ✿

Celebrating Our Green Mission – May 22, 2009

Dear KP Colleagues,

We only have one planet. It's lovely, but it needs our help. We need cleaner air, fewer fossil fuels burned, and we need to preserve and protect our water.

Last week, I wrote about our greener National Quality Conference. That was one more step in a long journey. Kaiser Permanente decided to be "green" several years ago, and we continue to figure out green things to do in every part of what we do.

We have been building green buildings, using green energy when possible, reducing our chemical waste levels, and taking steps to share our learnings about green caregiving with other health care institutions.

We are far from perfect, but we are making progress in a number of areas.

We now use about 40 percent less water per hospital bed than the national average. And we still use an average of 107,143 gallons of water per bed per year.

We have significantly reduced the number of harmful chemicals involved in the medical imaging and scanning process by going primarily to digital imaging.

We use a huge number of monitors, screens, desktop and laptop computers in our care sites and offices. Last year, all newly deployed equipment within KP earned at least a "silver" rating by the Electronic Product Environmental Assessment tool.

We recycled 74,000 pieces of KP electronic equipment in 2008 — rather than dropping them all into landfills.

In Northern California, we recycled nearly 100 percent of the demolition waste from our new San Leandro site and 97 percent of our packaging waste from our Modesto site that opened last year was recycled.

In Southern California, we are testing out new prescription bottles that are made with recycled materials — materials that studies have shown reduce the carbon footprint of these containers by 60 percent. We are also testing new biodegradable mailer bags for our prescription mail order facilities.

We are looking at ways to be greener all over our organization, because being green is clearly the right thing for us to do.

I am mentioning our achievements in my weekly letter this week because we just won another environmental award. The "Practice Greenhealth" national environmental safety and stewardship awards were announced on Tuesday of this week at the CleanMed conference. We won the "System for Change" award for our leadership in improving environmental performance in the health care sector.

CleanMed 2009 is actually a global conference for environmental leaders in health care. They gave us the "system" award for eco-friendly practices as a system.

On a more local level, twelve of our facilities and regions also won the "Greenhealth Environmental Excellence" awards from "Practice Greenhealth" at the CleanMed 2009 Symposium.

We continue to co-chair the Global Health and Safety Initiative — a coalition of major health care organizations across the industry who want to learn from each other about how to deliver optimally green health care.

The important thing for us is not to win awards for being green. The important thing is to be green.

We are greener now than we were a year ago — and we are not as green as we will be a year from now.

One last point — we decided a couple of years ago that any time we can have our patients eating local food, we avoid the negative carbon footprint that comes from flying, trucking, bussing, or literally shipping food in from overseas. Local food is usually just a little greener than the food that has major transportation elements involved in getting it to us. In addition to our 30 nationally recognized farmers markets — where we help both KP employees and patients get access to healthy and organic local food — we now have more than 25 of our hospitals serving locally grown food to our patients.

Better food and less carbon.

I have personally been to only one of our markets. I go to the one in Oakland. It's worth the trip. I can say absolutely that some of the best fruit I have ever eaten in my entire life came from that market. The food at that market continually exceeds my expectations. As a side benefit, I usually enjoy talking to the people who actually grew the food. Their pride in that great food is good for the heart.

If you have a KP farmers market nearby, my advice is don't miss the opportunity to eat really well. And encourage local farmers.

This week's letter isn't about the food. It's about the award.

Congratulations to our care site folks who are green enough to have us receive the Practice Greenhealth national award for systematically helping to protect our environment.

It's a good award to get.

Thriving comes to mind.

Be well. Stay well.

George

✿ ✿ ✿

Celebrating Our Greenness – May 30, 2008

Dear KP Colleagues,

This is the right time to be very green. We only have one planet and one environment, and we need to do everything we can to preserve and protect both for ourselves and our kids and grandkids and for everyone who will come after them.

To date, we have made a lot of mistakes — most from ignorance and scientific naiveté. We haven't protected our waters or the air we breathe anywhere near as well as we should have.

But those are the cards that have been dealt, and so we need to figure out now what to do next. I mentioned in an earlier weekly letter that we were doing some significant green work in our major building projects. We are now accelerating that work — and we have started a national coalition of health care organizations to share information about both green building and green operations. That organization is called the Global Health and Safety Initiative. Other member health care organizations now include Ascension Health, University of Chicago Medical Center, Catholic Healthcare West and St. Joseph Health System of Orange. Partnering organizations include the American Nurses Association, the U.S. Centers for Disease Control and Prevention, and the U.S. Environmental Protection Agency. We are currently on a recruiting campaign to bring other major health care entities into this shared learning cooperative relative to environmental sanity.

We have a great deal to share. National Facilities Services has documented 196 ways our building designs and standards protect safety and the environment. KP is making this information publicly available through the Global Health and Safety Initiative in order to enhance the performance of the entire health care sector. KP's cost per square foot for our new buildings built to these standards is nine percent less than industry benchmarks in California. Safety, sustainability and affordability can be achieved simultaneously.

Consider patient controlled analgesia (PCA) pumps and sets. Procurement and Supply is contracting for new PCA pumps and sets that are totally free of polyvinyl chloride (PVC) to eliminate dioxin pollution.

These new devices will cost 10 percent less than our current contract, and will promote marketplace transformation to safer products.

We also have begun to do some work with our own staff — urging green purchasing, green energy use, and even green eating.

We have programs to encourage use of canvas shopping bags rather than plastic or paper, for example. You can get KP fabric bags at the KP brand store.

We also are encouraging the people of Kaiser Permanente to be personal frugal energy users. The energy savings that would result if each of us simply used one fewer light bulb per day could be significant. I personally try to have one light bulb less at home every day, and we only turn on the lights in my office space in Oakland at dusk or on dark days. My windows provide enough light for the kind of work I do. That is not true for most of our workspaces, so I am not suggesting that other people do what I have done, but it does work well for me. We used to turn the lights on in my office automatically every day at the start of the work day. Now we don't.

I first experienced using window light only in Uganda when I was working on micro health plans there. None of the Ugandan offices turned electric lights on during day light hours except in the rainy season. It didn't take very long for me to adjust to using just natural light, but it was an adjustment that I did not initially appreciate.

In any case, we need to encourage people to use less energy — to use metal instead of disposable plastic water bottles where appropriate, and to ride share or use public transportation when available.

We also need to continue to set examples for our greenness — and that is what I am celebrating this week. Two weeks ago, there was a global conference in Pittsburgh, Pennsylvania, called CleanMed 2008. It was an international conference for environmental leaders in health care.

We won twelve awards at that conference — for our various projects to reduce waste and prevent pollution.

We won one award, for example, for eliminating 630,000 grams of mercury from our system over the past several years — leaving us 95 percent mercury free. This is just the beginning. We have a lot further to go. But it is a good beginning, and it's a path we continue to follow — getting smarter and more effective as we go forward.

So congratulations to the people of Kaiser Permanente who did the green projects that resulted in those twelve awards.

Well done.

Be well.

George

☆ ☆ ☆

Celebrating Our Contributions on Earth Day - April 22, 2011

Dear KP Colleagues,

April is the month when the CleanMed people grant their national awards for organizations in health care who prevent pollution and reduce waste.

We just won 17 of those awards.

Some of our green projects are so innovative that they are making news all by themselves. We started a purchasing scorecard system, for example, that rates the products we purchase by their environmental impact.

Our new standards and our scorecard for smart purchasing are becoming models for the rest of health care. We introduced that scorecard last year and met with a half-dozen major health systems to offer it to them. More than 130 media outlets ran stories about our scorecard.

We are continuing to improve that process and we just issued scoring system number two to build on our first efforts. The Kaiser Permanente "Generation II Sustainability Scorecard for Purchasing Medical Products" is now available to other purchasers and several tell us they are beginning to use it.

We also just announced a revolutionary deal to buy 12 megawatts of solar power from Recurrent Energy in an arrangement that will have them put solar panels on the roofs of 13 of our buildings and then sell us the electricity from our roofs at a reduced rate.

That deal created waves of interest at the World Economic Forum in Davos because it was a new alignment of green and business efforts that might possibly create a new business model for very local green power. More than 250 news media outlets did stories about our solar panel arrangement.

We also just entered into an arrangement with Bloom Energy to provide another five megawatts of power from fuel-cells at seven of our California facilities by the end of this year. Fuel-cells also have their advocates and deserve a good test.

It isn't clear yet exactly what combination of green energy-generating approaches will be the best for either us or the country. We are using our purchasing power and our site control to test and pilot several vendors' approaches. We are doing that because pioneers in that field need real customers to prove or disprove their technologies and their business model. We need electricity. We buy a lot of electricity. We are a real customer. We want to support the green generation of electricity. So it makes sense for us to be pioneer customers for innovators to help "prime the pump" for that level of innovation.

We also are continuing our efforts to be greener recyclers of our own various waste materials. We now recycle 31 percent of our total waste volume, preventing that waste from going to landfills. Our Colorado Region is a star performer with more than 50 percent recycled waste.

Fifty percent sounds like only half way — but in comparison with other organizations who recycle, it is a huge success. The greenness contest run for the country by Practice Greenhealth — another environmental advocacy organization — gives their top achievement award to organizations who average 24 percent recycling.

Even our farmers markets create a positive green impact that goes beyond much of the food being literally green. It's a good package. Green food grown in green ways. We are now up to nearly 40 farmers markets in various KP sites. The markets have great food. I shopped in one on Wednesday. I ended up with bags of magnificent dried cherries and some fresh pears that were tree-ripened to the point of perfection. The food from the farmers markets has a much lower carbon footprint impact because it doesn't have to travel 2,000 miles to get to our mouths. Food that travels can't be tree-ripened because when the food is grown on the next continent, it is a very long way from the tree.

We are also buying more sustainable food for our hospital patients and our care sites. We set a goal for ourselves of buying 15 percent of our food from sustainable sources by 2012. We actually hit that goal in 2010 — two years ahead of schedule.

We reprocessed over 164 tons of medical devices last year.

And we responsibly resold or recycled over 73,000 pieces of electronic equipment last year as well.

Our IT organization has also done excellent work to set a multi-year plan for "Environmentally Preferable Electronics." That plan will be a model for the industry, and has also won awards. The Uptime Institute just gave us an energy efficiency award that went to Microsoft and Google in prior years.

We have reduced demand by a 1.4 megawatt sustainable energy cut. We also reduced carbon dioxide emissions by more than 5,500 tons, an equivalent to taking 1,370 cars off the road annually.

We are also reducing our own exposure for our KP caregivers and patients to PVC, DEHP, and various persistent bio accumulative toxins.

We have done pioneering work already in those environmental exposure reduction areas.

We intend to continue that work and get even better at it.

Green is fully in our spotlight and on our agenda. We only have one planet. We need to use it carefully and well. We need to protect our environment and we need to protect our people and our patients from dangers that can spill into our environment.

For health care, our goal continues to be — to be the Queen of Green. If you have questions or ideas about how we can be more green, check out our interactive KP IdeaBook Green Community site.

So my letter this week celebrates our green team — all of the folks who work consistently every day to figure out how we can be continuously green and help the world around us be green.

And my letter celebrates the 17 green awards that we just won this month for our green health care successes.

Well done.

Be well.

George

☆ ☆ ☆

Celebrating Our IT Win – November 11, 2011

Dear KP Colleagues,

Green is good.

Computers take a lot of electricity. Computer centers actually take a huge amount of electricity.

We use computers to support care at multiple levels, and we have a lot of computers.

So being a good steward of the energy use of our computers is a very good thing to be if we want to help protect our environment.

That's our plan and that's our goal — to be a leader and a pioneer on green IT.

So how are we doing in that regard?

Computerworld magazine just rated the top 12 environmentally responsible IT organizations in the country.

They rated companies in multiple industries on green IT. They evaluated practices and approaches that reduce waste, reduce carbon dioxide emissions, minimize energy cost, and limit the use of toxic chemicals.

Twelve companies made their best company list.

We won.

Number One.

We not only made the twelve-best list, Computerworld rated us the best major organization in the IT world for green IT practices.

Being the best is a good thing. It did not happen by accident. We were both practical and creative. We built innovative cooling systems. We worked on a whole range of heat and electricity efficiency programs. In the process, we also earned an incentive award from our local power utility for optimal energy conservation practices.

One of the innovations that caused Computerworld to rank us number one for Green IT included inventing and using a new index — the CRFE. The "Computer Room Functional Efficiency" index is a new way to measure cooling efficiency in data centers. It's a measurement approach created by our data center facilities group that lets us figure out how to cool each of our computer rooms and use less power at the same time. The new CRFE metric also won the Uptime Institute's 2011 Green Enterprise IT Award.

Our facilities group also designed and implemented customized Computer Room Air Handling Units. These units blow filtered air through our hardware, cooling the air, and then circulating the air back into the rooms so we don't have to keep using and cleaning new, unfiltered air.

That common sense approach turns out to be very green.

Our facilities group also retrofitted some of our machines with common sense "smart" fans that continuously monitor room temperature and adjust their speed accordingly. We very carefully sealed air leaks throughout the computer rooms, and we were able to shut down several cooling machines that were no longer needed because we conserved cool air.

Cooling is a process that uses and sometimes wastes a lot of energy.

The air in our data center is cooled with water that is circulated throughout the facility and then run through an electric "Chiller." Chilling water is an expensive, power-intensive process. Our facilities group brought in a new machine — a water temperature economizer — that also utilizes water that has been naturally cooled outdoors during the winter months. Again — common sense and creativity are a nice combination. Using cool, outside air to cool water lets us bypass the power chiller for some of our water and use Mother Nature as our refrigerator unit.

These innovative changes are very important processes that keep us on the right road to protecting our natural resources, our environment, and ultimately our health and the health of our patients.

We were actually the only health care organization in the world that made the top-twelve Green IT list.

We have been on a good track for IT awards in recent weeks. In addition to the top green award, we also won the continuous availability award for our main data sites from the Uptime Institute.

The Uptime Institute recognizes large data centers that have continuous operational availability for years on end.

The Institute just announced this year's list of winners. No one else in health care delivery has ever received an Uptime award. We received three last year and we received four this year. Altogether, we've won 10.

This year was a clean sweep for our data sites. All four of our national data centers now have won the Uptime award.

The European Union is currently looking at how to optimize use of computers to support care delivery in Europe. They just had KP information in the center of the spotlight for some discussions in Brussels — looking at how we use computers to support care delivery and improve care.

The European Union is looking at us because we are delivering great care to nine million people as well as doing great research, and because we are leading the way on care connectivity for both patients and caregivers.

Europe is also trying very hard to be green.

When the European Union folks learn that we are also winning awards for having the best green program for IT and the environment, I suspect their respect for us as a truly responsible organization will continue to grow.

So my letter this week celebrates our green team — keeping KP on track to be the queen of green — and it also celebrates our operations folks who keep our data centers humming.

The number one rating is nice.

It's good to be the best.

Be well.

George

* * *

Celebrating KP, the Queen of Green – October 12, 2007

Dear KP Colleagues,

So what are we celebrating this week? KP as the "Queen of Green."

Last week, the U.S. Environmental Protection Agency and the Green Electronic Council named Kaiser Permanente a "Green Electronics Champion." Kaiser Permanente is the first and only health care organization that the EPA has honored with this award for "going green."

This week, the Journal of the American Medical Association (JAMA) held Kaiser Permanente up as an example of how green building and purchasing practices can have a positive impact not only on health care but also on the U.S. economy.

Those are just the two most recent examples of how green we are.

So how green are we?

We're pretty green.

Our organization actually has deep green roots. Four decades ago, we invited Rachel Carson, author of the groundbreaking book "Silent Spring," to Kaiser Permanente to deliver a seminal address to a large group of our physicians and scientists. Her powerful book — which exposed the hazards of the pesticide DDT - has been widely credited for launching today's environmental movement. We promoted that book at that time, because we believed healthy people needed a healthy environment.

Our actions have followed in that pathway ever since. We should celebrate our greenness.

We have led the way in green building, environmentally responsible purchasing and "sustainable operations." By sustainable operations, I'm referring to our deliberate and on-going efforts to divert waste from landfills, eliminate mercury from our health care operations, and end the purchase and disposal of hazardous chemicals. Our mercury elimination projects set the standard for our entire industry.

It is important for us to be leaders in environmental stewardship.

Health care facilities in the United States generate nearly five billion pounds of waste per year that pose occupational and environmental threats. In addition, health care accounts for 11 percent of all commercial energy use in America and is a major water consumer. Because of the intensity of our energy use, the US health care sector is the second largest contributor to carbon dioxide pollution, a greenhouse gas that causes global warming.

Our recent achievements in each of these areas are sizeable. In the past 5 years, for example, we have chosen ecologically sustainable materials for 2.7 million square meters in new construction. We have prevented the release of 70 billion pounds of air pollutants each year. We have saved more than $10 million per year through energy conservation strategies. And we have installed more than 50 acres of reflective roofing.

Our organization is also improving our communities' carbon footprint by supporting local farmers. We promote healthy local food by sponsoring 38 farmers' markets around the country. We are piloting the use of local fruits and vegetables on a seasonal basis to our patients in Northern California. This year, we will buy 50 to 60 tons of healthy food that is local, pesticide-free and farmed using sustainable methods. It's another great learning opportunity for us. We plan to expand that program in the years ahead. Our members and our communities will benefit.

Major media outlets and leading environmental groups have recognized Kaiser Permanente for our green leadership. Stories about our green building, sustainable food policies and environmental achievements have appeared in the Wall Street Journal, Newsweek and on NPR, among many other publications and broadcast outlets.

We have received quite a few awards for our greenness. I mentioned the one we received this month. We also recently became the first health care organization to earn the distinction of "Climate Action Leader," when we agreed to publicly report our 2005 and 2006 greenhouse gas (GHG) emissions with the California Climate Action Registry. The Los Angeles chapter of Physicians for Social Responsibility gave us the Socially Responsible Medicine Award earlier this year for our green successes and Hospitals for a Healthy Environment (H2E) gave a "Making Medicine Mercury Free Award" to 24 KP medical centers in California.

These programs have not been accidental. We work at it. In 2001, Kaiser Permanente leaders came together to form an internal Environmental Stewardship Council and to provide a framework for incorporating environmentally responsible practices across the organization.

The collaborative effort to be green has been especially timely and powerful because we are in the midst of multiple building projects. That gives us a lot of purchasing leverage. We are investing approximately $24 billion in 4,000 current and upcoming construction projects between now and 2014. For these projects, we will be following 176 environmentally-friendly design standards as we aim at building some of the greenest medical facilities in the country. We are able to do this and still have our construction costs about 5 percent below the industry average.

A prime example is our Modesto Medical Center, which earned national recognition this year as one of the greenest health care construction projects in North America. Solar panels on top of the Modesto Medical Office Building (MOB) produce electricity and pump it back into the grid, generating enough energy for 10 to 20 homes. The parking lot there is paved with permeable asphalt, which allows water to percolate through the surface and recharge the ground water table. This prevents flooding. Because it eliminated the need to connect to the local waste water management infrastructure, it also saved $290,000. Green can be very win-win when smart people take it on as an agenda.

Going green often makes good business sense. Like the switch to permeable asphalt in Modesto, we're seeing that many of our environmentally friendly changes are actually helping us "Bend the Trend." Another example is our elimination of mercury from medical facilities. Because we led the way in finding viable alternatives to mercury, we avoided the risk of mercury spills. These spills can run at a cost of $250,000 per incident. That's not including any medical treatment for exposure to mercury.

We're also saving roughly $300,000 per new medical center by replacing PVC pipe with safer HDPD (polyethylene). PVC, or polyvinyl chloride, is a dangerous and environmentally-unfriendly plastic material that is used widely in the health care industry. When manufactured and disposed of, it creates dioxins, the most potent carcinogens known, as well as other compounds that may cause severe health problems, including cancer and birth defects. We deliberately make construction choices that do not use PVC. We also set a new national standard for environmentally safe hospital carpets — and managed to get manufacturers to change production specifications because we can buy in such volume.

Those taking care of patients in our medical centers are also making a huge difference. For example, as we replace our traditional x-ray equipment with digital imaging machines, we're reducing both toxins and greenhouse gases. We just take x-rays for granted as a fact of medical life. What people don't think about is the fact that processing x-ray film uses very corrosive chemicals. The film itself contains silver, a toxic heavy metal. We're also saving water and energy that was used to dispose of these water-polluting chemicals. By doing digital imaging rather than x-rays, we expect to save over 154 million gallons a year of potable water just because we don't need all of those chemicals for processing our images. We have already converted Northern California and Southern California is following suit as we speak.

On October 17, we will be helping to share our green learning with other health care organizations as we launch a new collaboration called the Global Health and Safety Initiative that aims to improve worker, patient and environmental safety. We'll be joined by senior leaders from major health systems, leading non-governmental organizations, government agencies and Group Purchasing Organizations to discuss specific ways we can, together, advance health care's contribution to creating a cleaner and safer environment.

I personally have been a member of the Sierra Club, Greenpeace, The Wilderness Society, Nature Conservancy, and a number of local "green" organizations for years — so when I was looking at Kaiser Permanente as a place to work, Kaiser's long-time "greenness" was a major draw for me.

We are not perfect. We make mistakes and we have our missteps in various places — but our overall level of greenness goes right to our sense of who we are and what we do.

We want everyone to Thrive. It takes a healthy environment for that to happen. So think green. Turn off unneeded lights. Avoid unnecessary energy usage. Look for opportunities to make a difference. If you haven't seen Al Gore's movie, get a copy and watch it. It's a message we all need to take to heart. This is the only planet we have.

So be well — and be green.
Let me hear from you.
George

* * *

Background Note: We Want Healthy Members and Healthy Employees – And We Want Everyone to Walk

We want a healthy planet. We also very much want both healthy members and healthy employees. We are a health care organization. We are also an organization committed to health. We see that combined role as a dual responsibility. We want to deliver the best care, and we are also committed to improving and even optimizing health... for our members and for our patients.

We have become committed to an approach to health that is clearly anchored in "HEAL" — Healthy Eating and Active Living.

Both eating and activity are extremely important.

We know that most chronic diseases are caused by behaviors. We know that 75 percent of the cost of care comes from people with chronic conditions. We know that chronic conditions are caused by behaviors. We know that when people eat healthy food and are physically active, the rate of chronic diseases can be cut in half.

We also have come to understand that the single most effective pathway to better health for most people is actually activity — with walking very high on the positive activity list.

Walking can have an almost magical impact on the health of many people. The human body is clearly made to walk and functions better in many ways when people walk.

The Lancet — the official publication of the British Medical Society — just published a wonderful 80-page report showing that inactivity is a bigger problem for the world and kills more people than obesity.

We know that science and we understand that reality. We have been building that knowledge into our own agendas for several years — and we are learning how to do it well.

The next several letters celebrate our commitment to improving health by increasing activity levels. The first letter summarizes why we are using walking to anchor much of our health improvement agenda.

Everybody.

Walk.

Celebrating Reinforcements in the Effort to Walk Our Way to Better Health – August 24, 2012

Dear KP Colleagues,

A couple of years ago, we took a very practical look at various ways that we could help improve the health of the people we serve. We concluded that the single most effective thing we could do to improve health was to get people to walk.

Most chronic conditions are caused by two behavioral factors — unhealthy eating and inactivity. We have put a lot of effort into helping people deal with the issues of being overweight and being obese. Those efforts are the right thing to do, and they will continue.

But we also know that inactivity can actually be a greater risk for people than obesity. New science tells us that the health risks for totally inactive people equal or exceed the health risks for people who are overweight.

We also looked at comparative risk numbers of affected high-risk people. Those numbers were shocking. We learned that even though more than 30 percent of the American population is obese, more than 50 percent of the population is functionally inert — with very low activity levels.

Being inert is a bad and dangerous thing.

The human body is made to walk. Our bodies need to walk to be healthy. People who walk 30 minutes a day, for five or more days per week, are half as likely to be diabetic, and 30 to 40 percent less likely to have heart attacks, stroke, or several kinds of cancer. Breast cancer, colon cancer, and prostate cancer all happen at significantly lower levels in people who walk.

We learned that walking those same 30 minutes a day that can cut the rate of diabetes in half also has a major positive impact on depression for many people — with the benefits of walking exceeding the benefits of antidepressant medication in a couple of studies.

So knowing all of this to be true, Kaiser Permanente started down a road to get our own members, our employees, and even the communities around us to walk.

We put up a website to support walking. We developed a walking support app. Links to both are at the end of this letter. We held a walking summit for senior health leaders and media people in Washington, D.C., and — in our own Center for Total Health in Washington, D.C., next to Union Station, we even built a "walking wall" — a 40 foot long interactive video display panel that teaches people who interact with the wall about the benefits of walking.

We also added activity levels to our electronic medical record as "a vital sign." We may be the first major care organization in the world to make that addition to its electronic medical record. We created walking prescription pads to encourage activity increases for our patients.

We even had 40 caregivers walking alongside our float in the Tournament of Roses Parade this year to show how important walking is to our care team.

That walking parade unit got a huge round of applause at one point in the parade when a young woman watching the parade collapsed in the street, and our caregivers rushed to her rescue. I heard that people who saw her collapse were yelling, "It will be okay. Don't worry. Kaiser Permanente is here."

We actually had the original cast of The West Wing TV show do a very funny pro-walking video that has had a huge number of YouTube viewings.

So we have been promoting walking in a very significant way for a very long time.

So what am I celebrating this week?

We are now not alone. We have reinforcements.

The world is beginning to join us in our understanding of the need for increased activity levels and the wonderful potential for walking.

The Centers for Disease Control and Prevention — the CDC — just held a national press conference and announced that physical activity is truly a wonder drug. The CDC said that walking is a great way of improving health. The director of the CDC said that "walking will reduce your risk of getting high blood pressure, cancer, and a host of other conditions." That was a direct quote.

The leadership of the CDC now clearly sees that improving activity levels through walking is a top priority for American health.

WE WANT HEALTHY MEMBERS AND HEALTHY EMPLOYEES

Across the Atlantic Ocean, the British medical journal, The Lancet, just put out an 80-page report saying that inactivity was a damaging and destructive worldwide epidemic that kills many millions of people every year.

The Mayo Clinic also just issued a press release saying that improving activity levels is crucial to population health.

Even Dr. Oz, the noted TV medical personality, recently issued a statement that calls walking "the single best thing you can do for your health."

The experts are coming to understand how important activity levels and walking are to everyone's health — as a global issue.

We are more convinced than ever that our walking agenda is the right thing to do. All of the data tells us that we are on the right track.

New science shows that sitting and being totally inactive is highly dangerous to our health.

So my letter this week celebrates the fact that other health care experts are becoming converts to the cause of walking. We have been teaching, preaching, and supporting walking agendas in multiple settings. For a fairly long time, we were almost alone. But we were right — and when you are right, being alone is an okay place to be — as long as we help other people learn why we have come to believe what we believe. When we do that teaching well, learning happens. Learning how to improve health is a very good thing.

So thank you to all of the care teams at Kaiser Permanente who are helping our own members walk. And thank you to all of the people at Kaiser Permanente who are now personally walking. We improve our own personal health when we just get up on our own two feet and when we each make 30 minutes of our own day special for our own health. Doing the walking in two 15-minute periods seems to work as well to improve health as one 30-minute walking period. A lot of people at Kaiser Permanente knew that to be true, and a lot of us are now making walking part of our daily lives.

So thank you for walking.

And thank you to the health care research community who keeps adding more supportive data points on the benefits of walking until the total mass of evidence in favor of walking has become overwhelming.

Now we need to help show all of the new converts to walking all the things that we have been learning about how to facilitate and support walking in the workplace, in schools, and in our communities.

We have done some good work in each of those areas. It's time for us again to share what we have learned — and for us to keep on learning. We are far from perfect, but we are having an impact, and we are getting growing numbers of people to walk.

Well done.

Be well. And everybody — walk.

George

Every Body Walk!

Every Body Walk! App

✧ ✧ ✧

Celebrating Walking, Good Times, and Better Health – January 14, 2011

Dear KP Colleagues,

It is time to celebrate walking.

There are very few things that we can do that have a more positive impact on our health and our lives than walking.

Walking feels good. Walking cheers people up. And walking has an amazing array of positive results when it comes to our health.

Studies have shown that walking 30 minutes a day, five days a week, can cut new cases of Type 2 diabetes by nearly half.

Our bodies are made to walk. Walking gets the blood flowing through our veins, and changes our blood chemistry to increase the percentage of good (HDL) cholesterol in our bodies.

Walking briskly for 30 minutes a day can reduce the risk of stroke by 25 percent. Walking can also have a positive impact on depression. People who walk report a lower level of depression. One very credible study of women who were depressed and started to walk showed that the women in the depression control group who did not walk had a Beck Depression Inventory (BDI) score of 13.5 points at the beginning of the study, and they still had a score of 12.5 points at the end of the 12-week study.

The women who were depressed and walked, however, had their BDI scores improve from an average of 14.81 at the beginning of the study to only 3.27 by the end of the 12-week study. That is a huge difference.

Another study showed that when people between the ages of 60 and 65 walked on a regular basis, they had a significantly lower risk of developing both cognitive impairment and dementia.

Reducing the risk of dementia is a good thing.

Walking definitely helps prevent heart disease. People have known that to be true for a long time.

What people didn't know to be true until recently was that walking helped patients recovering from certain cancers survive longer. No one quite understands why this might be true, but the studies seem credible and the results seem clear. For prostate cancer, one study showed that

383

patients who walked 90 minutes a week had an almost 50 percent lower mortality risk. Another study showed that for women recovering from breast cancer, regular walking reduced the relative rate of both recurrence and mortality by about 50 percent. Walking also seems to reduce the risk of colorectal cancer.

Our bodies clearly function better when we have walking as a regular part of our lives.

Another entirely unexpected benefit from walking is that it can help prevent the common cold — and another credible study done at Appalachian State University reported that people who walked benefited by having their cold symptoms for as much as 46 percent less time than non-walkers who also had colds.

Again, no one really understands all of those benefits or why they happen.

The researchers from the cold symptom study theorized that walking makes the blood flow faster, so it is possible that increased blood flow brought the body's natural immune system cells to each of the actual virus sites more often.

Over time, very smart people will figure out why those benefits exist.

Is it better to run or walk? That has been a topic of debate over time. People take both sides. What we know to be true is that both are extremely beneficial to our health, but walking is generally much easier on the body. Walking a mile and running a mile burn about the same total number of calories. All of the health benefits that I just mentioned are triggered by walking. So walking works as well as running, and walking does less incidental damage.

Walking tones muscles and makes them leaner and more efficient. Walking also can create feel-good chemicals — endorphins — in the brain.

An ideal health package would be a combination of healthy eating and physical activity. Healthy eating and eating in moderation are both very good things to do, and they do improve health.

Our HEAL agenda for years has focused on two themes — Healthy Eating and Active Living. We have long sponsored healthy eating campaigns and we have created a whole array of great farmers markets for healthy food — and now we will try to get everyone to walk. Active living is possible and it can feel very good.

Walking has great benefits — whether done alone or as a part of a package of healthy behaviors.

Walking can create a very consistent positive and beneficial outcome relative to our personal health — and, the really good news is, walking generally feels good.

Walking often creates a very nice set of experiences. We can walk in groups. Walking can be very social. We can walk to explore and we can walk to learn.

I love walking through neighborhoods and cities because I see the world around me much better and more completely than the world I see when I just drive by in my car.

Walking has given me the gift of my town.

Walking is a good thing.

So my letter this week celebrates both walking and the new work that Kaiser Permanente will be doing to help people walk.

Kaiser Permanente is on a new path, so to speak, to encourage everyone in America who can safely walk, to walk.

The theme is — Every Body Walk!

We already encourage "walking school buses" for kids in several of our communities. Kids very much need more walking time. We have helped fund walking paths in a number of neighborhoods. We have supported a bunch of community walking programs. We want to support walking — and we want everyone to walk.

So what is our new walking program?

Dr. Bob Sallis, the former president of the American College of Sports Medicine, is a 25-year Kaiser Permanente physician who will be our national medical spokesperson for the new Every Body Walk! campaign.

Dr. Sallis practices in our Rancho Cucamonga clinic in Southern California. He has been prescribing walking for his patients for decades. He is a nationally known expert on walking. He has done important research on the linkage between walking and health. Dr. Sallis is a passionate advocate for walking as a prescription for better health.

Dr. Sallis is featured in a series of videos about walking — walking and diabetes, walking and heart disease, walking and depression, etc. We will be putting those videos and our Every Body Walk! support information on the Internet next week, and we will be promoting them at no charge as a public service to community leaders and to communities across America.

You will be able to see the videos next week at www.everybodywalk.org.

It's the right campaign for us to do. Every Body Walk! is the logical and natural next step in our Thrive agenda. Our videos show communities that have become walking friendly. The videos show kids walking to school in "walking school busses." The videos show people who love to walk talking about why they walk.

So watch the new videos next week. Check out the website. Recommend it to friends. If you have a friend who is at risk of becoming diabetic, you can be a great friend to your friend by getting your friend to watch our new video piece on diabetes and walking. It's an amazing piece.

And, whenever it makes sense, walk.

One of the very best new pieces of science about walking is that 30 minutes a day achieves almost all of the goals and — even better — we now know that the 30 minutes can be done as two 15-minute increments. That is super information. We don't have to do all 30 minutes of walking at once. Two 15-minute walks have the same health benefit. That is great news because it can be hard to find a full 30 minutes to carve out of our busy days — but it is usually a lot easier to find two 15 minute times. Fifteen minutes in the morning and 15 minutes at night get the job done. Or 15 minutes instead of a coffee break. Or 15 or 30 minutes of walking during a lunch break. In any case, it's a good idea to find 15 minutes and walk. And then do it again later.

My letter this week celebrates the new Kaiser Permanente program to get us all to walk.

Walk on.

Every Body Walk.

Be well.

George

☆ ☆ ☆

Celebrating Every Body Walk! Week – October 7, 2011

Dear KP Colleagues,

We sponsored a walking week in Washington, D.C., a week ago. The United Nations held their first time ever summit that week in New York City on the topic of chronic disease. We held our own summit at that same time in Washington, D.C., focusing on how to prevent and alleviate chronic disease. Our summit featured walking as an achievable, workable, functional, easily accessible way of bringing down the rate of chronic disease and helping patients who suffer from chronic diseases.

We brought in local, national, and international experts on the multiple benefits of walking — scientists, physicians, epidemiologists, therapists, and public health policy experts — to share an array of extremely important data about the links between walking and health.

We also organized mall walkers, park walkers, and people who walk to work every day, to make the point that walking is entirely possible to do in the real world.

As prep for the walking week, I videotaped a script about walking.

It's an interesting script. I liked the script so much, in fact, that I have included the exact walking talk script at the end of this letter. That script makes some fascinating points about the benefits of walking.

Every data point in the script has a scientific study behind it. All of the data points and research references are available on our walking website — Everybodywalk.org.

I am including that script here for two reasons. One is that I do like the script a lot and want to share it. The other reason is that I am very curious about how people respond to that particular array of data points. I, personally, find that set of data points to be fascinating and persuasive — but I want to learn their impact on other people.

So I am in learning mode as I write this letter. I would like to try an experiment. I need help to do the experiment. Please consider reading the actual script at the end of this letter out loud to a friend, a family member, a coworker, a colleague, or a neighbor.

Read it to them, and then ask for a reaction.

Then send me a note telling me how the person responded. Were they shocked? Were they delighted? Were the points convincing? Was there a hole in the argument? Was there something missing? Did the data points seem important or not important? Did the person you read it to pay attention and have some level of interest all the way to the end of the script?

And here's a key question:

In the end, after hearing the points, do you think the person you read it to is more or less likely to actually walk? Did the script cause the person to say, "Hey — I should actually walk"?

Let me know. And let me know how the points could be improved.

My letter this week celebrates all of the KP folks who put on and hosted the really well done Walking Summit at our new Center for Total Health in Washington, D.C. Our new center is a great place to do that kind of meeting. Real learning and real teaching happens there.

It was a good summit. People learned a lot about walking.

You can see a highlight video from the Walking Summit at our Center for Total Health website.

And if you do read the script below to someone, let me know how well or how badly the script and the key points were received.

Thank you.

Be well.

George

The "Benefits of Walking" Video Script

The human body is made to walk.

Our bodies function better when we walk. We are healthier in many ways when we walk.

Walking 30 minutes a day cuts the rate of people becoming diabetic by more than half — and it cuts the risk of people over 60 becoming diabetic by almost 70 percent.

Walking cuts the risk of stroke by more than 25 percent.

Walking reduces hypertension. The body has over 100,000 miles of blood vessels. Those blood vessels are more supple and healthier when we walk.

Walking cuts the risk of cancer as well as diabetes and stroke.

Women who walk have a 20 percent lower likelihood of getting breast cancer and a 31 percent lower risk of getting colon cancer.

Women with breast cancer who walk regularly can reduce their recurrence rate and their mortality rate by over 50 percent.

The human body works better when we walk. The body resists diseases better when we walk, and the body heals faster when we walk.

We don't have to walk a lot. Thirty minutes a day has a huge impact on our health.

Men who walk thirty minutes a day have a significantly lower level of prostate cancer. Men who walk regularly have a 60 percent lower risk of colon cancer.

For men with prostate cancer, studies have shown that walkers have a 46 percent lower mortality rate.

Walking also helps prevent depression, and people who walk regularly are more likely to see improvements in their depression. In one study, people who walked and took medication scored twice as well in 30 days as the women who only took the medication. Another study showed that depressed people who walked regularly had a significantly higher level of not being depressed in a year compared to depressed people who did not walk. The body generates endorphins when we walk. Endorphins help us feel good.

Walking strengthens the heart. Walking strengthens bones. Walking improves the circulatory system.

Walking generates positive neurochemicals. Healthy eating is important — but dieting can trigger negative neurochemicals and can be hard to do.

Walking generates positive neurochemicals. People look forward to walking and enjoy walking.

And research shows that fit beats fat for many people. Walking half an hour a day has health benefits that exceed the benefits of losing 20 pounds.

When we walk every day, our bodies are healthier and stronger. A single 30 minute walk can reduce blood pressure by five points for over 20 hours.

Walking reduces the risk of blood clots in your legs.

People who walk regularly have much lower risk of deep vein thrombosis.

People who walk are less likely to catch colds, and when people get colds, walkers have a 46 percent shorter symptom time from their colds.

Walking improves the health of our blood, as well. Walking is a good boost of high density cholesterol — and people with high levels of HDL are less likely to have heart attacks and stroke.

Walking speeds up metabolism and burns calories. Walkers often find that eating habits change and weight loss results from those eating changes.

Walking significantly diminishes the risk of hip fracture — and the need for gallstone surgery is 20 to 31 percent lower for walkers.

Walking is the right thing to do.

The body needs to walk.

We don't need to walk a lot — 30 minutes a day makes the body work better.

The best news is that the 30 minutes doesn't have to be done in one lump of time. Two 15 minute walks achieve the same goals. Three 10 minute walks achieve most of those goals.

We can walk 15 minutes in the morning and 15 minutes at night and achieve our walking goals.

Walking feels good. It helps the body heal. It keeps the body healthy. It improves our biological health, our physical health, our psychosocial health, and helps with our emotional health. Walking can literally add years — entire years — to your life.

It's good to walk.

Be good to yourself.

Be good to your body.

If you can — where you can — walk.

Everybody.

Walk.

Be well.

George

✿ ✿ ✿

Celebrating The West Wing Walking – May 4, 2012

Dear KP Colleagues,

It is a very funny feeling to look at a computer screen and see Martin Sheen — playing the President of the United States — saying some of the words from my own video script on walking.

The cast of The West Wing had a secret reunion a couple of weeks ago to film a public service announcement for Every Body Walk!. They all generously donated their time.

Allison Janney does the voice-over for many of our Thrive messages, so it was also a bit strange to hear the "Voice of Thrive" talking about how the country should create a "Walking Agenda."

The video is great fun. It definitely promotes walking.

Walking works. Walking 30 minutes a day, five days a week cuts diabetes in half — helps relieve depression — and reduces the rates of several cancers.

I am attaching my own video walking script again to the end of this letter. As you may remember, I used that script last year to record a statement for our websites about the benefits of walking. Look at that old script and then watch The West Wing video.

We gave the script to The West Wing crew as input for their video. Martin Sheen used part of it in his presentation. Fun to see. Here is the link ⤢.

The West Wing piece had a third of a million viewers in the first four days of its release. We will add it to both of our walking websites — Every Body Walk! and KP Walk!.

So my letter this week celebrates the folks from our Communications team who helped the "Funny or Die" crew get The West Wing walking again.

Well done.

The old walking video script that Martin Sheen looked at is attached.

Be well.

George

* * *

Celebrating KP Walkers and the Every Body Walk! Mobile App – January 13, 2012

Dear KP Colleagues,

We started this year with 28,900 walkers participating in walking programs at Kaiser Permanente.

That is, as near as I can tell from looking at a couple of reference points, the largest number of walkers for any organization in the world.

The second largest company with a walking campaign has about 10,000 walkers. That particular organization has about 80,000 employees — so we beat them both on total walkers and percent of walkers.

Our walking float in the Tournament of Roses Parade created a bunch of media attention — with several national news media fascinated by the fact that we have caregivers so committed to walking that nearly 50 walked the length of the Rose Parade route to make a point about putting our feet where our message has been.

We walk because walking is one of the very best things we can each do for ourselves. We walk to be healthy. I have written earlier letters about the fact that walkers are much less likely to become diabetic or have strokes or get some types of cancers.

The health benefits are invaluable, but many of us walk for other reasons. Many of us walk because walking makes us feel good.

Feeling good is a good thing. Depression levels are lower in walkers — and people who are depressed and walk have — on average — a significantly higher likelihood of reducing their depression — but that also isn't why most of us walk.

We walk because walking feels right and because there are so many side benefits to walking that the side benefits outnumber the primary benefits.

I have traveled to a lot of cities. They are more interesting when I walk through them. I see the streets and neighborhoods and people in ways that I completely missed when I used taxis and vans and tour buses.

And my own community is now much more immediate to me. I know about buildings and houses and side streets that completely passed me by when I passed them by on wheels.

Walking around the San Francisco Bay is a joy. Lake Merritt here in Oakland is lovely. All of our cities have places to see that only get seen when we are on our feet and have the perspective to see them.

So we walk for our health, and we walk for the sheer pleasure of the walk.

So what am I celebrating this week? I am celebrating two things. I am celebrating the fact that the total number of "unduplicated" KP walkers for KP Walk! and Thrive Across America reached 28,963 people for 2011 — and I am celebrating another new app.

We have given the world a nice new mobile app to encourage, support, and reinforce walkers.

The app is called — not surprisingly — the Every Body Walk! mobile app.

It helps with walking routes, tracks walking times and places, and encourages walking.

It's free.

Hopefully, it will help encourage people to take a walk. The walking app has been very well received, and it is already rated number five in the list of top 100 green apps. That's a good sign that it may be helping people.

So thank you to the team who put the app together and who keep the app up and running.

And congratulations to the 28,963 people who walked in the last year.

A year from now, I hope that number will be even higher.

Be well. Stay well.

George

* * *

Background Note: Healthy Eating and Reducing Obesity Are Important Agendas as Well as Walking

Walking isn't the only tool in our health improvement toolkit. We also are working very hard at multiple levels on healthy eating. In fact, earlier this year, we were a co-sponsor with the National Institutes of Health for the major multi-star HBO documentary series, "The Weight of the Nation."

Any time we can help people with healthy eating and any time we can help a patient deal with the issues of obesity, we are doing wonderful work. We need to keep getting better at doing that work. We need to help our patients and our communities with healthy eating knowledge and capability.

The next letter celebrates both our sponsorship of The Weight of the Nation and our total commitment to healthy behaviors in some measurable ways.

Celebrating The Weight of the Nation and our BMI Quality Scores – February 10, 2012

Dear KP Colleagues,

Chronic diseases are primarily caused by behaviors.

We all know that to be true.

The number one cost driver in American health care is now chronic diseases. More than 75 percent of all care dollars go to buy care for patients with chronic conditions.

So what behaviors cause chronic diseases?

The two primary drivers for chronic conditions are obesity and inactivity. We have been working hard to deal with both concerns. We have been dealing with inactivity by helping our patients and our members and employees to walk. Walking has an amazing ability to reduce the rate of chronic diseases, including diabetes and heart disease.

A new study indicates that walking even has a very strong, positive impact on protecting the brains of people who are genetically at high risk of Alzheimer's. A link to more information on this study is worth reading.

So walking is on our radar screen and we are dealing with activity levels at KP in a number of increasingly effective ways.

We are also devoting quite a lot of energy to dealing with all of the issues relating to obesity.

Our Healthy Eating Active Living (HEAL) campaign and our Total Health strategy have both been focused on helping our people become healthier.

So how are we doing relative to those goals?

NCQA — the National Committee for Quality Assurance program — measures how well health plans do in a couple of dozen areas of performance. Because obesity is such a huge problem for America, one of the NCQA quality measurement areas relates to health plans helping patients keep track of BMI — body mass index. BMI is a good thing to measure, track, and talk to patients about if we want to help people manage their weight.

So how are we doing in the annual NCQA BMI national health plan performance scorecard?

We are the best.

Kaiser Permanente has the number one plan in the entire country for BMI measurement for Medicare patients. Georgia wins for the entire country.

So how did our other regions do?

We also had the number one ranking regionally in Washington, D.C., Maryland, Virginia, Colorado, Oregon, Washington, Hawaii, and Ohio.

In California, we were number one and number two.

So the only state where we ranked number two on BMI measurement was the state where we beat ourselves by also being number one.

We need to help our members with issues of weight and obesity. We have a wide range of programs and educational resources to do exactly that — including helping to set up farmers markets in a number of our care sites and communities.

Until recently, our efforts on obesity issues were fairly local and our work was primarily linked to each of our care systems. We are now going national.

We have been helping the first lady with her national agenda to help kids with healthy eating and active living to reverse childhood obesity in one generation. We have provided expertise and some funding to support that effort. People from Kaiser Permanente were at the White House when that program for kids was announced two years ago, and people from Kaiser Permanente have been there since to celebrate its progress.

Childhood obesity is also a major problem for this country. NCQA is also, therefore, concerned about the weight of children and also uses the HEDIS (Healthcare Effectiveness Data and Information Set) scorecard to measure how well health plans do relative to pediatric BMI measures.

So how did we do for kids?

Not surprisingly, we also had the highest scores in the country on the NCQA childhood BMI measure. Our Northwest Region was the number-one plan in the nation for kids.

Now we are going one major step further down the road of helping people with obesity. We are helping HBO produce a series of extremely powerful programs that we hope will teach the entire nation about obesity. The documentary series and the public health campaign that will accompany it are called The Weight of the Nation.

We are doing that obesity work in very good company. We are working with The Institute of Medicine (IOM), Centers for Disease Control and Prevention (CDC), and the National Institutes of Health (NIH) to develop and promote that program. The support team for the series has been those government agencies, plus two. We are one of the two. Kaiser Permanente and the Michael & Susan Dell Foundation (MSDF) are the only non-governmental members and sponsors of The Weight of the Nation obesity education team.

We have been helping our partners think about how to engage the country about this huge problem.

The series will be on the air in a couple of months, and then we expect that it will be replayed thousands of times in schools, workplaces, community organizations, and clinical settings.

We hope that the teaching and the stories from that HBO television program and The Weight of the Nation campaign will help Americans understand obesity and deal more effectively with issues of weight and healthy eating.

So that's what I am celebrating this week...our number one HEDIS scores in the country for BMI measurement of both our Medicare patients and kids, and our Weight of the Nation partnership with HBO, IOM, CDC, NIH, and MSDF to engage America and share truly important information about one of the major health issues of our generation.

Again, we are doing good work that needs to be done.

Well done. Thank you.

Be well.

George

* * *

Background Note: We are Encouraging Healthy Behaviors for Our Own Staff as Well

An earlier letter mentioned the fact that we now have nearly 30,000 registered walkers inside Kaiser Permanente. One of my weekly letters celebrated the fact that our Kaiser Permanente float in the Tournament of Roses Parade this year was a huge floral walking caterpillar — and it was surrounded by 40 physicians and nurses walking the entire parade route to demonstrate our commitment to actually doing what we preach. Our healthy workforce agenda means a lot to us — and we are getting healthy activities built into our culture and our expectations for how we deal with the world.

We need to help the people we serve increase their activity levels. The employers and government agencies who entrust us with their employees and beneficiaries deserve having us help both employees and beneficiaries improve their health.

We have started with our own employees. We just won the platinum award for best practices for a healthy workforce from the National Business Group on Health. I celebrated that platinum award with a letter that is not included in this book.

I have written a couple of letters celebrating our total health agenda. This letter triggered a lot of good responses because it helps explain the worldwide explosion on chronic diseases in very practical terms. A number of our folks told me that was very useful information.

Celebrating Our Healthy Workforce Initiative – April 30, 2010

Dear KP Colleagues,

Diabetes is becoming the number one disease in a whole number of countries where it used to be extremely rare.

Why would that happen? Diabetes isn't caused by a germ or microbe. It also isn't biologically contagious.

So why is it growing so rapidly in so many places?

The answer is simple. Simple and sad. Diabetes is a disease of inactivity and unhealthy food.

I was at a meeting with the CEO of one of the largest diabetic supply companies in the world this January. They are a Swedish company.

He told us that diabetes is a "disease of urbanization" — and when people move from the countryside to the cities in any country, the number of diabetics explodes.

Why?

In the countryside, people walk. In the cities, they either ride or just stay in their own confined neighborhood and sit. Urbanized people walk a lot less.

They also eat different food. Processed white rice, processed sugar, and processed wheat products replace fruits, vegetables, grains, nuts, and very lean goats and chickens.

So people are inert and they eat less healthy food — and the number of diabetics has tripled.

Diabetes is also the fastest growing disease in America. We are on a path to have half of the kids in school today becoming diabetic by their mid-forties.

That is a really ugly projection. We owe it to ourselves to make sure it does not come true.

That's why Kaiser Permanente is doing farmers markets, improving meals, and educating students about Healthy Eating and Active Living in schools. It's why we have sponsored biking and walking paths in several communities. We have a number of community activity projects underway.

It's also why we partnered with First Lady Michelle Obama last month to pioneer the new national initiative to reduce obesity in children.

We are trying to educate our members about how to avoid diabetes. It can be done. We can clearly do it. Walking 30 minutes a day five days a week cuts the number of new diabetics by 40 percent — and then if people lose 10 pounds and also walk, the number of new diabetics can be cut by almost 60 percent.

Medicare would be saved financially if we cut the number of new diabetics by just 40 percent.

So we are telling our members and our patients to eat healthy food and be physically active.

That's for our members.

What are we doing for the people who deliver care and work at Kaiser Permanente?

Until now, we have done about the same things for our own staff that we do for all of our members — good things that do help people.

We are now increasing those efforts significantly.

We have decided to crank our own internal health agenda up a bit for our folks and we have set up a new online health improvement program for our staff. We have had success with similar programs in NCAL and Colorado so we know they work.

Our Healthy Workforce team calls this next step "Thrive Across America."

We are suggesting to all of our people that we should form teams in our work sites to encourage physical activity levels — with the symbolic goal of "walking" from our east coast regions to our west coast regions — with team members supporting each other as a team and — if anyone feels competitive — competing with other teams.

I have joined together with my co-workers to form a team. I will personally be doing the "Thrive Across America" walk. I had been a good walker until I hurt my knee on Minnesota ice a couple of years ago — spent several months on crutches — and then never got back to consistent walking.

I do need to walk. So this is very much the right thing for me to do — and I can now do it with a team who will be supporting each other in the process.

Our preliminary team name is the "Chair Steppers." If anyone has a really good idea for our team name, let me know. We will vote on the best ideas.

So we will start walking next week. We won't be walking alone. Since the overall program was announced last week, nearly 9,400 KP staffers and over 600 teams have signed up to exercise and Thrive Across America.

It's not too late to sign-up and explore all of the features from the Thrive Across America Website.

So this week I am celebrating the Healthy Workforce team who created "Thrive Across America."

If even one of us doesn't become diabetic, that is a huge win.

And good science shows us that walking also reduces the risk of heart disease, stroke, and a couple of cancers — so the side benefits could be a really good thing.

Be healthy.

Be well.

And walk.

George

✻ ✻ ✻

Background Note: If You Smoke, Please Stop – And Please Never Smoke Again

Almost no personal behavior does more damage to people than smoking. Smoking is a very debilitating and personally destructive behavior. As part of our Total Health Agenda, we also very much want people to stop smoking. We want our members, patients, and staff members who smoke now to stop smoking. Smoking is the single most damaging behavior that large numbers of people do to impair their health.

Inactivity and obesity create a lot of chronic diseases problems and need to be addressed. Both of those conditions cause health to deteriorate. But for individual patients, the behavior that causes the most direct and personal health damage is the act of smoking.

Smoking is amazingly damaging. We need to help people who smoke stop smoking, and we need to help people who do not smoke avoid smoking.

We do have a wide range of anti-smoking approaches. Some of those approaches were celebrated in the next letter. This particular letter triggered an avalanche of emails from our staff that sent notes agreeing with the points in the letter and telling me their own stories about smoking for themselves and family members.

One of the letters I received from one of our staff members told me about his father who was dying of emphysema and who asked for a final cigarette literally with his last breath.

So this letter is focused on the issues of smoking and giving up smoking.

Celebrating Our Work to Help Our Members Stop Smoking – May 13, 2011

Dear KP Colleagues,

My father smoked.

He averaged nearly two packs of cigarettes a day. The addiction of smoking brought him emphysema and then a massive heart attack.

He did not live to age 60. One of my great regrets in life is that my own sons did not get to spend time with my father. Cigarettes stole those years from him and from all of us who cared about him.

We can do really good things to improve our health. We can walk regularly — and that can significantly reduce the risk of heart disease, stroke, diabetes, and even some types of cancer.

We can eat well — healthy and nutritious food — and we can avoid artery clogging, carcinogenic, highly unhealthy foods — and that can also have a huge positive impact on our longevity and our lives.

The single most effective thing anyone can do to improve health probably is — however — to stop smoking if you are a smoker.

Smoking kills. Smoking makes every major disease worse. Smoking makes people less attractive and much less healthy.

Helping people who smoke stop smoking is the single most effective thing we can do to improve many people's lives.

We know that to be true. We are, at our heart and our essence, a care system — a collective of people who are working together at Kaiser Permanente to improve people's health and deliver great care.

For smokers, health improvement can begin with giving up that addiction.

It isn't easy. My father stopped smoking several times. What he did not know is that the addiction never goes away. The constant, consistent, continuous, and intense craving almost always goes away after roughly a month — a miserable month for many people — but the good news is that the craving always does eventually subside, and the addiction then takes a nap. It doesn't go away. It just naps a bit — a little like a screen saver on a computer — and then, when you smoke again, the screen saver

407

disappears and the addiction jumps back on screen and the addiction takes over people's lives again.

My father did not know the danger of a single cigarette or any type of nicotine to reactivate the addiction when the cravings were finally napping. So when he would quit and be craving-free for a bit, it seemed safe to him to have just one more smoke.

It never was. The addiction is an addiction, and addictions will nap but they never disappear.

My father didn't know about screen savers, and we lost him way too soon.

So what are we doing at Kaiser Permanente about tobacco use for our patients and our members?

We are working hard to help people quit. We include smoking as a vital sign on our electronic medical record. Our goal is to encourage smokers to quit at multiple clinical encounters.

We offer counseling, classes, and various health education programs. We provide services in person, by phone, and online. We help members to design personalized plans to quit smoking.

We encourage members to use an online HealthMedia program called "Breathe" — and that program has a 59 percent average quit rate — but only for the 7 percent of our smokers who responded to the Breathe survey.

We have various programs that also involve tobacco cessation drugs. We believe those drugs work best when combined with behavioral modification support. In some cases, we require the modification support as a condition of making the drugs available to patients.

The most effective way for people to stop smoking and then successfully continue to not smoke is the oldest approach — to simply pick a day and then stop smoking entirely on that day. And then never, ever, ever, take into your body anything that restarts that addiction cycle.

Cold turkey is really hard. It takes anywhere from three weeks to two months for the tobacco cravings to go on screen saver status — and that can be a really hard several weeks.

Some people who are going cold turkey think the cravings will last forever — and they break the cold turkey rigor after a couple of miserable weeks to have just one cigarette. That one cigarette, unfortunately, just starts the clock all over and then achieving the cravings "nap cycle" is delayed because there is a full restart to the whole process. That is sad and extremely frustrating. Many people give up at that point — sometimes very near to the point where the cravings would have gone into remission if they had just lasted a while longer.

We need to help people stop smoking. We also need people to understand that once the cravings and the addictive desires go to full screen saver status, one nudge of the nicotine mouse can restart the old addictive programs in our brain.

So how are we doing at KP in helping smokers quit? Our best results are in Southern California. In 2007 we had an 11 percent smoking rate. We are now down to under 9.5 percent.

That is encouraging progress.

The Consumer Assessment of Healthcare Providers and Systems (CAHPS) program scores health plans on three categories of smoking cessation support. Plans are rated on advising smokers to quit, discussing cessation medications with patients, and discussing smoking cessation strategies with patients.

How did we do on our CAHPS scores compared to other health plans in California?

Interestingly, we were near the very top of the list on advising smokers to quit. We were very high on discussing smoking cessation strategies.

We were also high — but we were not leaders — on discussing the use of smoking cessation medications with patients.

That last score — medications — makes some sense as a more moderate score for us because we provide smoking cessation advice to patients based on the needs of each patient and that particular score assumes that it is always the right thing to do to think of medications as an option for all smokers.

Medications are, in fact, clearly less desirable if people can go cold turkey and stop smoking. Medication is a path to use if cold turkey fails or isn't an option.

We know medication is the right approach for many patients but not for all patients.

So what do we know about smoking?

Smoking kills.

Smoking ruins lives.

Smoking can be avoided — and people can be helped to stop smoking.

My own father smoked a morning set of cigarettes the day his heart failed.

I really wish that someone had been able to help him learn to manage that addiction to nicotine. I wish that someone had warned him about the fact that the addiction never goes away — and one cigarette can re-trigger the cravings. I wish he could have been with us longer.

So my letter this week celebrates all of our people who work in so many ways to help smokers stop smoking.

It is good work to do. It is important to do it well.

Be well.

George

✿ ✿ ✿

Background Note: We Have Reduced Heart Attacks By A Lot

Overall, we have had a positive impact at Kaiser Permanente on the health of many people. We are committed to that agenda of Total Health — and that agenda has a lot of moving parts. Some work very well.

Our healthy eating programs and improved activity programs were described in earlier letters in this book. Our walking agenda has been increasingly important and effective.

We also are doing important things in the context of traditional care delivery — managing the medical risks in very medicinal ways.

Our hypertension programs, for example, may be among the most successful in the world. For HEDIS quality scores, we tend to lead in areas like diabetes care and prevention. We tend to win in performance areas like mammograms and cancer screenings.

We are constantly trying to figure out how to use our entire toolkit to change the trajectory of diseases so that our patients have fewer crises and fewer traumatic care events.

We have been successful in that work in multiple areas. A number of my letters have celebrated those successes.

The next letter is one of those celebrations. Reducing the number of heart attacks is a very good thing to do. Total health is better when heart attacks don't happen.

Celebrating Our Heart Health Progress – June 11, 2010

Dear KP Colleagues,

One of our major objectives is to help our members be healthier.

Great care is good. Being healthy enough to not ever need great care is even better.

Our goal is to help our members benefit from both of those realities. We have a whole series of things we do to achieve both goals. Our heart surgery success levels, for example, are among the highest in the country.

That is something to be deeply proud of.

And we also should be proud that we are doing things to help a lot of people not need those heart surgeries.

How are we doing on those prevention programs? We are far from perfect, but we are doing fairly well. More than 200 newspapers just wrote stories about the fact that our focus on the heart health of our patients has reduced the total number of heart attacks for Kaiser Permanente patients significantly. For our Northern California heart patients, for example, over the past decade, we have reduced total heart attacks by almost a quarter — and we have reduced the rate of the most serious heart events by more than 62 percent.

We also significantly reduced the death rate for the patients who still had heart attacks.

As someone who had a heart attack followed by a quadruple bypass surgery a couple of years ago, I can tell you very directly and clearly that being opened up, repaired, resealed, and then rehabilitated is a whole life experience that is not at all pleasant in many aspects, and it was definitely levels of care I would have been very happy to have been able to avoid.

I had great surgery. I very much needed that surgery. It was not, however, pleasant and the rehab was — particularly in the very early stages — its own level of misery. That's one of the reasons why I am such a strong supporter of walking today — because I don't want to be doing my walking again in rehab. (Our walking team is in 662nd place right now — by the way. Moving up.)

Heart attacks are not good to have. So when we say that we have reduced serious heart attacks by over 62 percent for our members, I personally celebrate that success from the heart. It may just be a data point for some people, but it makes lives better in very real ways for quite a few very real people.

The New England Journal of Medicine published the study about our reduced heart attacks this week. You can read about it on their Website.

What did we do?

We helped patients lower their high cholesterol, control their blood pressure, and lose weight. We used a lot of heart health medications in the process. We provided team care for our heart patients.

Planned, systematic, patient-focused care works. Prevention and great focused care make a great package.

As I mentioned, more than 200 news outlets ran the study. We were a major story on TV shows like the CBS Evening News and CNN, and other major media like National Public Radio and WebMD.

In these days, when inactivity and obesity are increasing the heart health risks for huge numbers of Americans across the country, the news media found us to be a bright spot in the health improvement universe. We are a bright spot.

Thank you to the care teams who continue to make our care improvement and health improvement successes real.

Be well. And walk when you can.

George

☆ ☆ ☆

Background Note: We Also Want to Be Good Stewards, Members, and Citizens of Each KP Community

We exist to make a difference for our members, for our patients, for the employers and government programs who buy our care for their people, and also for the communities we serve. We make that difference for our members, patients, and customers with great care, great science, continuous learning, and a real commitment to people's health. We do most of that work directly as an organization.

We also do some important work in communities individually as volunteers.

We encourage our staff members to personally be volunteers in ways that will help other people in their communities. I write a letter each year celebrating our employees who take the time to make a personal difference in their communities. We have a lot of people doing very good things. These good things are worth celebrating.

The next two letters celebrate some of those efforts. One of my goals in writing those letters about people who volunteer is to encourage additional people to volunteer. I have no data on that point, but anecdotal feedback tells me that a number of people are at least considering going in that direction based on the inspiration of some of the people whose efforts and successes I celebrate in these letters.

Their efforts inspire me every year.

I also love writing those letters about our volunteers and our community support efforts.

Celebrating Community Service – September 26, 2008

Dear KP Colleagues,

This week I am celebrating nominations.

Every year, we give an award for community service. We ask for nominations from our employees and staff. We ask for the names of people or programs who have made a major contribution to their communities as a pure public service — work done out of a sense of stewardship, service and giving. You can see write-ups on the winners for the last couple of years on our Community Benefit Website.

This year, the awards committee had a really challenging time picking the winners because there were so many great nominations. We had nearly 300 nominees to choose from.

It was an impressive list. The committee had a very hard time selecting the award winners.

We will announce the actual winners in December — with a dinner held next Spring to present the actual awards.

What I am celebrating this week is not this year's winners — but the rich stream of nominees.

So what kind of nominations did we receive? I love the list.

We have people who created and founded free clinics. We have people who do animal rescue and care. We have volunteer counselors for children with congenital heart disease. We have nominees who created a domestic violence prevention and intervention program for the local Asian-American population in one of our cities.

We have people who do voluntary rehab for the homeless. We have people who set up cross-cultural competency programs and other people who set up volunteer medical care for homeless shelters.

We have folks that do air search and rescue, and we have people who do voluntary community mental health counseling.

It is a truly inspirational list.

We have clinicians who provide the voluntary care for a battered women's shelter. We have people who work with community stroke victims and other people who provide counseling to pregnant teenage girls. We have people who volunteer for healthy eating programs and healthy living programs and who run anti-tobacco programs. We have people who provide transitional counseling for community people who need support groups.

Volunteering is a very special way to spend time. Everyone I know who volunteers says that they get back more than they give — because it feels so good and so right to really make a difference.

We are basically caregivers, so large numbers of our staff have the blessing of being able to make a real difference in people's lives every day at work. In addition, we have large numbers of people who go on to make a real difference in people's lives after work, on weekends, and on vacations.

Those are the folks I am celebrating this week — all 272 people who were nominated for this year's David Lawrence Community Service Award — and an equivalent number of people who were nominated the year before and the year before that.

I will get to thank the winners in person at the award dinner early next year. For now, in this letter, I want to thank the entire list — all winners — who were nominated for this year's award.

Thank you.
Be well.
George

* * *

Celebrating All of Our David Lawrence Community Service Award Nominees – February 19, 2010

Dear KP Colleagues,

Two weeks ago when I celebrated our David Lawrence Community Service Award winners, I promised to mention some of the other nominees who were nominated for the award.

I really enjoy looking at the total list of nominees every year. We have people doing a lot of interesting and very valuable things for their communities. Some of that work is done through our organization. Most of it is done through volunteering efforts.

We have a number of physicians who are providing medical care and training for other health care professionals in developing countries. Our volunteers go to a lot of places. People in Africa, Central America, and the Caribbean are benefiting from the ongoing volunteer efforts of our employees and physicians.

We have people who are working with school districts in many of our regions. The school volunteer work includes creating safer routes to schools, helping with student health issues, and helping to improve the health and well-being of children by teaching and supporting both better nutrition and more physical activity.

We have quite a few people who are helping our most needy community members. We have people who work to feed and clothe the homeless, and we have people who help get homeless people off the street and connect them with the local support systems that allow the homeless folks to get back on their feet and live independently.

We have folks who do air search and rescue. We have quite a few folks who drop everything and fly off to disaster-ridden areas in times of urgent need. Several of our doctors just did that last month to help the earthquake victims in Haiti.

We now have ongoing volunteer support efforts there.

We have volunteers from Kaiser Permanente who help with mental illness issues, and we have volunteers who help care for children with autism. We also have a number of people who volunteer to help and assist victims of domestic violence.

When I look over the total list of 180 nominees, I am reminded and encouraged by the fact that so many people from Kaiser Permanente are out in our communities every day helping make our communities better, safer, healthier, and more functional.

We take care of people for a living. We are a caregiving organization. Our day job is to be the care system that people can count on for safe, caring, high quality, and consistent care. And then we have people from Kaiser Permanente who reach past our day jobs as volunteers to make our communities better and to take care of even more people outside of our care system.

That is important work.

Volunteering is a very special thing to do. Important things will not happen or get done unless volunteers do them.

We have quite a few volunteers. Our awards committee had a difficult time selecting this year's winners from our 180 nominations. The truth is every volunteer is a winner when it comes to doing the right thing and making the world a better place to be.

So this week I'd like to thank our inspiring total group of volunteers who were nominated for this year's award, and I would also like to thank all of the folks at Kaiser Permanente who give back to our communities as volunteers every single day.

Thank you.

Be well.

George

☆ ☆ ☆

Background Note: We Also Try to Make a Major Difference in the Communities We Serve – Nearing Eight Billion Dollars of Benefit

We do want to be very good citizens in every community where we deliver care. We actually have an extensive community benefit commitment involving multiple programs, agendas, initiatives, and direct contributions. That set of activities has created over eight billion dollars in community benefits during the time that I have been writing these weekly letters.

We have educational programs, outreach programs, research programs, and community health programs. We make direct cash contributions to a thousand organizations every year. We also run our own programs that are set up to create community benefit and provide needed care to people who otherwise would not be getting that care. We even have a community benefit committee of our Board of Directors that meets as many hours as our finance committee and more hours than our executive committee.

We write an official report to the community every year highlighting the things we do to make a difference as community benefits. When that annual report to the community is released, I usually write a weekly letter to our own staff making the report available and celebrating some of the activities covered by our annual report to the community. Overall, as I noted, we have made more than eight billion dollars in community benefit contributions while I have been writing these letters. So these letters are also easy to do and fun to write. The next two letters celebrate some of our commitments to the communities we serve.

Celebrating Our Community Benefit Achievements – July 24, 2009

Dear KP Colleagues,

Our researchers published more than 700 studies last year. This is part of our promise to share our knowledge and expertise with the medical and scientific community.

Several of those studies received worldwide recognition.

We also began work on a human genome project that will expand the science of medicine and human biology in ways that other organizations can only envy.

We made health institute grants to 1,181 community organizations, and we sponsored intensive and extensive Healthy Eating/Active Living programs for 40 communities.

We set up 27 HEAL programs in 2007 — so that agenda continues to grow.

Our Educational Theater Program reached more than 557,000 children and over 120,000 adults last year as well.

More than 5,000 of our Kaiser Permanente employees and staff members volunteered on Martin Luther King Day in nearly 80 sites.

Enrollment in our "Charitable Health Coverage" program for low-income members increased to over 100,000 people last year.

We also set up the first "virtual school" so that health professionals from all over the world can learn from experts about patient safety and effective care.

We are doing safety net packages in several communities and educational support programs in several others.

Our total Community Benefit contribution for 2009 is extensive and growing.

I mention these programs this week because we have just Web-published our 2008 Community Benefits Annual Report. It's available online.

The programs I mentioned above are just a flavor of our full contribution. If you have a few minutes, pull up the report and get a sense of the kinds of things we are doing.

We exist to be of service. Our community benefits help channel some of the ways we serve.

It's a good list — and a good thing to celebrate this week.

So scan the report and join with me in celebrating Kaiser Permanente Community Service.

Be well.

George

✿ ✿ ✿

Celebrating Our Community Benefit Outreach, December 2, 2011

Dear KP Colleagues,

One point seven billion dollars is a lot of money.

We will exceed that number with our Kaiser Permanente Community Benefit programs for this year.

We have a wide array of ways of benefiting the communities we serve.

Our community benefit programs include free care and low-cost coverage for significant numbers of children, families, and individuals with low incomes.

We also make grants to community organizations. More than 2,500 community groups received Kaiser Permanente grants in 2010 — the year covered by our most current community benefit report.

Most of the grants were for the health of people in the communities we serve. Some were for walking trails, walking school buses, and safe walking events.

A few of the grants were made directly to the communities we are in — like the more than $10 million we committed to support the Oakland school system.

We support Healthy Eating, Active Living (HEAL) coalitions in more than forty communities. Those coalitions have become a national model for both other funders and the federal government.

Research was a major part of our community service agenda. We had more than 3,800 separate research projects at Kaiser Permanente last year — and those projects resulted in more than 900 published research studies, as well as giving us great internal knowledge about how to improve care.

Some of our research studies were featured in the news media and publicized across many countries — with Kaiser Permanente science changing caregiving across the planet.

We also funded an extensive program of educational theater — with talented actors presenting extremely informative educational mini-plays to a record 737,000 students during more than 2,500 separate performances in approximately 1,700 schools. Our community theater teams have reached more than 15 million audience members since the program was launched 25 years ago.

We also helped with the core funding for a number of safety net clinics and hospitals who take care of people in medically underserved communities.

And we educated health professionals — helping with programs that train nurses, med techs, and other health professionals. The number of medical students and residents trained in our medical education programs now exceeds 2,500.

We make grants and contributions every month. We usually tell the local communities about our contributions. This press release is a typical community announcement of a local grant made by KP.

Our 2011 numbers won't be available until early next year — but a copy of our 2010 Community Benefit Report is available online.

One of the things that make us unique at Kaiser Permanente is that we have a Community Benefit committee for our health plan and hospitals boards of directors.

Most boards have finance committees and most boards have audit committees. Many boards have executive committees. Very few boards have community benefit committees.

We do have that committee on our board, and every meeting has a full agenda of community benefit programs, functions, strategies, and activities. We believe that community benefit is too important to just be something we peripherally do as a side agenda with no board insight or involvement.

If you would like to learn more about our community benefit programs from last year — take a look at our most recent community benefit report. It's worth reading.

My letter this week celebrates Kaiser Permanente making the commitment to make a difference and to be a community benefit.

We want the communities we are in to be better places because we are there.

Great care is central to our agenda.

Education, research, grants, and safety net and community support programs add to our value, as well.

It's a good package. We are making a difference.

Be well.

George

✼ ✼ ✼

Background Note: The Final Comment

So that's it... 101 letters written to the people of Kaiser Permanente. The letters were fun to write. I learned a lot writing them.

If you are not part of the Kaiser Permanent family, I hope this set of weekly letters to our staff offers a flavor of what we are trying to do inside of Kaiser Permanente across a broad spectrum of the work we are doing.

One hundred and one letters is roughly a third of all the letters I have written. You can also read a complete set of all my weekly letters at kp.org/ceoletters if you want to read more about Kaiser Permanente. The letters at that site are simply listed in pure chronological order with no explanatory notes or comments, instead of being roughly grouped and teed up by topic as they are in this book.

After personally re-reading all of the letters from the last five years or so, I do think that they offer some insight into us inside Kaiser Permanente. KP Inside is a good title for the book.

We are who we are. For someone who doesn't know us, these letters should give a flavor or a sense of who we are. For someone who wants to study us and even learn from us, some of these letters might help tee up and explain some of the things we do that make us who we are.

Every letter is a celebration. I do love celebrations. Having the function and the role of celebrating something every week for more than five years has actually been good for my own learning and my own morale. I suspect that I will continue to write these letters until I turn the baton for my day job over to my successor. Writing them is too much fun to quit.

This book actually is its own macro-celebration letter — with me celebrating being able to write weekly celebration letters about Kaiser Permanente for more than five full years. It has been fun to do. So I will celebrate the personal joy of writing all of these celebratory letters as the final celebration note and as the conclusion for this book of celebration letters.

It's been a good thing to do.

Be well,

George

Table of Contents — By
Title of Each Letter:

Made in the USA
San Bernardino, CA
22 July 2015